The Mothering Journey

Raw and Real Stories of Motherhood

Kate Blakemore

MUM'S THE WORD

Mum's the Word – The Mothering Journey
By Kate Blakemore

ISBN: 978-1-0686758-0-5

Published by: Maud Ann Books
Copyeditor and proofreader: Siân-Elin Flint-Freel
Book and cover design by Michelle Catanach
Images by Carol Rossini

Dedication

I would like to dedicate this book to those that make this possible in every way:

Steve, my amazing partner, and dad to my amazing three children.

This book is also dedicated to them for providing the content – Gracie Mai, Lennon and Dylan.

Also, Mum, Dad, and my sister Lisa for supporting me to be the mum I am today.

Contents

A little bit of "Motherhood Magic"

Being a mum has been one of the most difficult jobs I have ever done and I am quite sure it will remain one of the most difficult jobs throughout my life. Many of you will have heard the phrase, "It doesn't get any easier." I am completely appreciating that now – it hasn't!

As a mum, I am sure at some point you have felt alone, even when surrounded by well-meaning people. There is so much pressure to be the perfect parent, I am telling you. However, I want you to know that the perfect parent does not exist. It is so easy to compare yourself to others when looking at social media, in magazines, and reading books – books telling you how it SHOULD be done. But what about the honest stories of how it really can be?

'A little bit of magic' summarises how this book is going to go!

I am not an expert and no one else in this book claims to be an expert. However, everyone in this book has been or is a mum. It is jam-packed with honest accounts and no holding back. This book is for mums-to-be, and mums on the mothering journey. I would love for this book to be the go-to book for all mums as they progress through the different stages of motherhood. As a counsellor and a mum myself, I know the power of 'I have been there'. I hope this book helps you as you go through the most challenging but enjoyable stages of your life.

So, let me introduce myself. I'm Kate Blakemore – Mum, partner, leader, friend, daughter, sister, counsellor and volunteer. I am sure you can relate to the many different roles that you are within a working week. I have been with Steve, my partner, for twenty-seven years (we've never made it down the aisle). We have three children together: Gracie Mai (born 2007), Lennon (born 2009) and Dylan (born 2012).

I became a mum at twenty-seven years old, and like for most mums, becoming a mum changed me in so many ways, both physically and emotionally. It took me years to adapt to being a mum. I had always been quite a free spirit mixed in with being ambitious; from day one, I felt that these qualities of mine had been lost, leading to many years of a difficult journey, all of which is explored in this book, along with the stories of many others. We will be sharing the stories of both the good and the not so good.

I am proud of my mothering journey. I feel this journey has defined me as a person and supported me to make *Motherwell Cheshire* the charity that it is now. I have never really told my story but feel it has its place in this book. Lived experience is powerful and I want *The Mothering Journey* to reflect the lived experiences of not only me but all mothers.

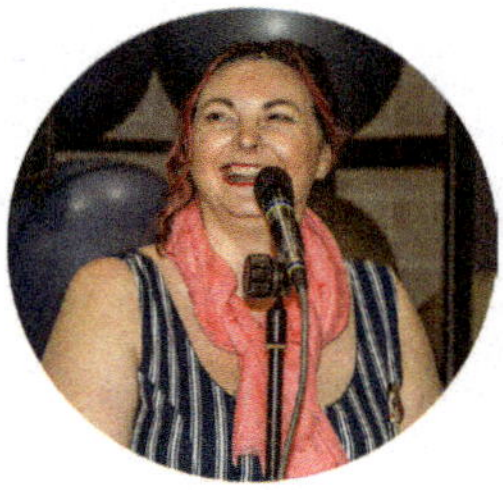

Kate Blakemore - Counsellor and CEO

Talking is my thing! Those of you that know me will know that I can talk! I love getting to know people; their thoughts, opinions and knowledge fascinate me. Ever since I was seventeen years old, I wanted to be a counsellor. The thought of enabling people to talk about their inner thoughts and feelings without fear of being judged really appealed to me. So as soon as I was old enough, I enrolled on a training course. As I write this book, I am entering my eleventh year of being a counsellor and love it today as much as I did in my first year. I feel so privileged to be a counsellor and to share the journeys of my clients. My specialist area is working with women, but in particular, mum's mental health. Although I have limited time now, with my other responsibilities of looking after the children, being a taxi, being a chair of a collaboration and swimming, I still run my private practice once a week. Although I am on a mission to make sure I find time for my relationship and me.

Ever since working in retail many years ago, I knew charity work was where my passion was, using my business skills but in a way that rewards every single day. I feel privileged to say that I am the founder of the charity *Motherwell Cheshire* CIO (*Motherwell Cheshire*), a women and girls' mental health charity. As I write this book, we are going into our tenth year and I could not be prouder of the amazing team that we are.

Setting up the charity was the next logical step for me after establishing my counselling private practice. I was getting so many mums contacting me for support but struggling to pay for sessions. I looked into setting up a not-for-profit strand of my private practice, and after talking to the right people at the right time, I was offered an opportunity that I couldn't refuse and the rest, as they say, is history. I can't believe where we are as a charity and the ambition in me will keep driving the charity forward to help support more women and girls when they need it the most.

Not only did the experiences of others lead me to creating *Motherwell Cheshire*, but also I founded the charity as I felt becoming a mum was the most difficult job that I have ever had (and continue) to do. I was fully supported by my family when I first became a mum, but at the time none of my friends had or were even considering having children, so in that way it was a bit of a lonely place. There were so many practical things that I didn't know, but soon found out by reading books and asking. My first child was a very easy baby and slept and fed at regular intervals. My second was very ill and I struggled to bond with him due to his time in hospital from being a newborn. However, we soon found our way, mainly through the support of my family and a great health visitor with whom I was able to have honest conversations.

However, I feel that the most important factor that helped support my mental health was that I was training to be a counsellor. From this experience, I had the opportunity to talk through what was going on for me in a safe and confidential environment. It felt safe to discuss the trauma of the birth of my second child, and also the issues of attachment and the struggles that I had/was having. Through this experience, I recognised how I was seeing situations differently and accepting what had happened.

This experience always stayed with me and when I had the opportunity to set up *Motherwell Cheshire*, I thought I would give it a go and offer a safe place for mums to come and feel comfortable in explaining their struggles. I have never regretted it, and as an organisation, we have grown and grown. This has proved to me that there was (and still is) obviously that need. Although *Motherwell Cheshire* is definitely not just for new mums, a big part of our work is supporting new mums. Many suffer from anxiety, depression, and some have postnatal depression. We deliver counselling and a six-week therapeutic course for new mums, complemented by wellbeing services. This approach has worked so far, and the feedback demonstrates that we have helped mums view themselves differently. Our focus is solely on mum, sometimes the forgotten party when a newborn comes along.

In a society that seems to have many parenting theories and a world in which social media is constantly showing 'perfect mums', I want to say there is no such thing as a perfect mum, only mums who are doing their best in very trying circumstances. Over the years, the charity has grown to be a well-established charity in Cheshire, supporting the health and wellbeing of women and girls. We are currently working on a name change for the charity to reflect our work now

Kate Blakemore, Author

I can't quite believe I am writing the word 'author', but I have wanted to write a book for a very long time! As well as a talker, I am also a thinker. Always thinking and reflecting on what I experience, read and research. Most importantly, I am always reflecting on what I hear from the amazing women that I come into contact with on a daily basis.

As I've said a couple of times already, becoming a mum was and still is the most difficult 'job' I have ever had and I wanted to write about my mothering journey as a therapeutic tool, for both you the reader and, I dare say, to myself. I then came up with the idea of capturing other mums' experiences and sharing them to help support others.

There are many books out there that are humorous, and these are great, but I wanted to capture real and relatable stories to help support other mums on the mothering journey. Being mum can be a very lonely place; so many mums can be alone with their children feeling they are failing. Mum guilt can be so relentless. It can take the joy out of being a parent.

The Mothering Journey captures all the emotions throughout the mothering journey, with the aim of supporting other mums on their path.

Kate Blakemore - Mary Poppins fan!

You will notice that there is a clear theme throughout the book – Mary Poppins! Ever since I can remember, I have loved the film. Everything about it makes me smile. The quotes, the songs, the style, and most of all, the two different stories that are taking place in the film. The magical side that takes us to fun places where we can escape and enjoy life, and the undertone of the film, about suffrage, inequalities and work life balance. It's simply amazing!

Throughout this book, I wanted to interject myself into it and thought there was no better way of doing so than using Mary Poppins as my alter ego! At times you will notice that there is a play on words as I don't have the time or the energy to take on Disney in a copyright court case!

I do hope you enjoy this book, and as our mission statement at Motherwell Charity states, I hope it Encourages, Inspires and Empowers every one of you.

A little bit of advice and guidance on the way.

Throughout this book, the contributors and myself will offer tips, **"A Spoonful of Love "**, and some guidance, **"A Sprinkle of light to lead the way"**. If you have any others to add to the mix, I would love to hear from you! There will also be reflections and helpful numbers and websites at the end of each chapter.

Today or never

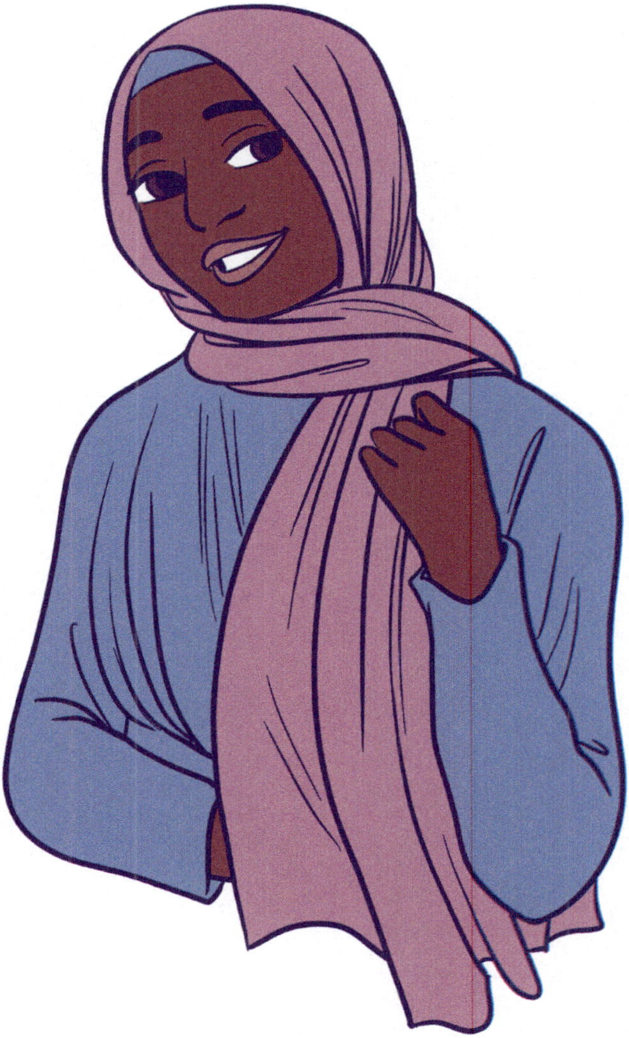

"Today or never" - When do you know it's time to become a mum?

I get asked this question a lot by women I have worked with, wanting to know if I think the time is right for them to start trying for a baby. The answer I always give is that it lies with the women themselves. It certainly wouldn't be for me to say. I am yet to find a definitive tick list that provides the answer to such a question.

Truth be told, none of my children were planned, but with each one of them I knew that I was ready. At the age of twenty-three I had an ectopic pregnancy, and it had only been twenty-four hours previously that I found out I was pregnant! At the time, I was upset about being pregnant because I knew that I wasn't ready. This sounds selfish but I just knew the time was not right. I was in a steady relationship but didn't feel ready for someone else to enter that relationship. I had a job that I loved and I wasn't ready to give that up. There were still many adventures that I wanted to go on.

Fast forward four years when I fell pregnant again, but things were so different. I was so happy about being pregnant and yet was scared stiff that I would lose the baby again.

Over the four years, not that much had changed in my life. I was still in the same relationship, but felt more stable. I had left the job that I had loved, but over time, as I became older, my priorities in life were changing and I was seeing my role at work in a very different way, questioning what I was doing all this for. Something had shifted and I was ready to embrace motherhood.

There are so many considerations when thinking about starting a family. It is very personal to individuals and couples, but here are some pointers that you may want to consider:

A Sprinkle of Light to Lead the Way – When is the right time?

There is so much to consider when thinking about trying for a baby, it can become quite overwhelming. Here are some areas that may be worth considering and discussing with others.

Support networks

Support networks are crucial when thinking of starting a family. This can be made up of friends and family, neighbours or your local community. All too often, I see women who, because they have no one to talk to, are struggling with their mental health. Not having someone to speak to and support you through the mothering journey can have a great impact on your wellbeing.

Financial stability

Financial stability is always a difficult one to discuss as this is relative to the person. Over the years, I have met many women who have wanted to become a mother with very different financial circumstances, which has proved to me that having money doesn't necessarily make you ready to be a mum, but financial stability is important – whatever that means to you.

What I do know is that living in poverty can greatly impact mum's mental health; national research has shown this and I see it first hand, running *Motherwell Cheshire*. I set up the charity to work in deprived communities to address this issue.

Employment

Linked with financial considerations can be employment, obviously for financial reasons but also for emotional reasons. Are you ready to either leave your job or take time off work? For many women now, a day's work plays a big part in their life, both career-wise and friendship-wise. This will change and can impact mental health and wellbeing in many ways: your sense of purpose, loneliness, lack of control. It can also have an impact on your career – unfortunately this can still be the case.

Being honest, I am not sure what I would have done differently but I do wish I had considered it more from the start, so it didn't surprise me and impact me as much as it did.

Support in the workplace

As I write this book, there is a lot of discussion at a national level about helping mums more to enter the workplace and in the workplace itself when they get a job. Here are some considerations that I have picked up along the way and that I try to put into place when leading a charity that has mums as part of the workforce.

- *Does your workplace have a flexible working policy?*
- *Is there an opportunity from your employers to help with childcare?*
- *Know your rights as a mum. There are many schemes in place that you*

may not know about: parents' emergency leave, right to taking annual leave, parental leave, etc.

- *What's your maternity pay? Do you need to have been working somewhere for a certain length of time before you can claim this? In the majority of cases, that's the case.*
- *Who are your 'friends' at work? It's important you have that safe space at work to talk through any anxieties that you have.*

Relationships

In modern times, many women are choosing to become a mum without a partner involved. However, where there is a partner involved, how strong is your relationship? Do you both want to become parents? Whatever you do, never have a child to patch up a relationship. This is the one time that I am going to be direct!

There is no doubt that starting a family has an impact on parents' mental health and wellbeing, which can add strain to any relationship. Lack of sleep, the full range of emotions that mums experience after giving birth, lack of libido, and priorities needing to change all take their toll. Different styles in parenting need to be considered and often don't get spoken about when planning for a baby. However, these are topics I see many couples struggle with in the first years and sometime beyond.

Linked with partners, friendships are also very important when starting a family. They can be your crucial support networks that I mentioned earlier.

"Listen to you – you will become the baby's mum no one else. Only you will know and feel when the time is right."

When I had my first two children, my closest friends were nowhere near considering having children, so I didn't have them to talk to, but also didn't have them to go out with, along with their children. As I was the first to have children in my friendship group, they didn't quite comprehend how my priorities had changed, sometimes asking me out to events that I didn't want to go to as it would have meant leaving my little ones for a long time, and that I wasn't quite ready to do. To be fair, they probably couldn't win because if I hadn't got asked, then that would have probably impacted me as well. A question to ask yourself is are you ready to make sacrifices like this? I'm not suggesting that you hold back on becoming a mother as none of your friends are yet mothers. However, you should consider how you will deal with the situation. Who will you rely on as your support network and is it possible to still spend time with your friends as a mother in a different way?

Practical considerations

There are many practical issues that you may want to think about. This book is based more on emotions so I don't want to go into them in detail, but you may want to consider the following:

Is your house the right size for a baby? A baby tends to come with lots of items.

Do you live in a catchment area of the school that you want your child to go to?

Will you be isolated from friends and family where you live?

How is your physical health? Would you be able to get pregnant? Carry a baby?

These are all considerations your GP would be able to support you with, but are important questions to ask.

This list can go on for practical points. My opinion is that in most instances, practical issues can be resolved, but emotional issues are not as easy to do so. Here other mums share their account of considering to be a mum.

My Journey to Motherhood – Emma's story

I think I have always wanted to have a baby. It is one of those things that I remember thinking about when I was little and when I was a teenager. It was one of those things that was almost expected of you, I suppose. But after my younger aunties and uncles had their children and I spent more time with babies and toddlers, I definitely felt like it was something I wanted in life.

But having a baby and wanting to be a mother are two quite different things. Seeing friends and family make the transition from woman to mother is a wonderful thing to witness. Their matrescence. (I love that word so much!) The changes are subtle and profound. On the run up to our wedding, one of my cousins had a baby. She was the cousin that I had always been closest to and seeing her change from my cousin to a mother was amazing. She took to it so well; the bond between her and her son was awesome and something in me changed.

Joe and I married in March 2012 and we had talked about starting a family soon after the wedding. But then the wedding happened and it felt scary all of a sudden. My mental health hadn't been great in the run up to our wedding. We had relocated from Rugby to Crewe the September before and I didn't feel very settled. I had moved so that Joe could be closer to his work as he had been commuting from Rugby to Stoke every day for nearly a year. I left a job that I loved, a lovely group of friends and a life that we were happy with. The move was the right thing for us as a couple but for me it was tricky. The job I moved to wasn't quite as good or enjoyable as I thought it was going to be. I had gone from having a good group

> and then after three months, two very faint lines appeared on a pregnancy test and my whole world changed.

of friends to not knowing anybody. Add to that the stress of planning a wedding pretty much all by ourselves and moving from a three-bedroom house to a tiny one-bedroom flat and I ended up in a bit of a bad place and was on anti-anxiety medication.

There were lots of doubts in my mind. A lot of worry that we were rushing to have a baby. Was this the right time? But would there ever be a 'right' time? The more we talked about it, the more it felt right. We might never feel ready with circumstance but we were ready and steady as a couple. We decided to stop using birth control. And after years of trying not to get pregnant, it felt weird to be not trying not to get pregnant – but it felt right. One month passed and nothing. Two months passed and nothing, and then after three months, two very faint lines appeared on a pregnancy test and my whole world changed.

"The right time" to have children - Kirsty's story

Everybody will have a different idea of when the right time is for them, to have children. Different factors will impact on your decision, and in many cases planning a pregnancy isn't always a simple timeframe.

Writing this, I'm thirty-seven years old and am six months pregnant with my first child. According to Statista, this is seven years above the average age of women having their first child in the UK in 2022. There's a clear upward trend in the average age of women becoming first time mums – in 1970 this age was twenty-six, in 2022 it's thirty. But I don't feel particularly old, it just feels like now is the right time for me.

So, which factors contributed to this being a good time for me? The first was probably very typical of what many women cite in the modern day – a sense of wanting to feel fulfilled in other areas of my life first. That is, feeling like I'd reached a point in my career which I was happy with before having children, and having travelled and visited places before the responsibilities of children set in. In honesty, I'm not sure that I'll ever reach a point where I'd not want these things, but I've certainly now come to a point in my life where I'm happy and excited to make sacrifices to aspects of my life, to welcome our child into the world. And I've also had the pleasure of speaking to so many parents with young children who have told me about the different joys of new experiences, like travel, since having their children.

> Lastly, and most importantly for me, I found the person who I knew I wanted to raise children with and who would be a loving and caring father to our child.

This brings me nicely onto a second factor – my age. If your planned pathway is biological children, then especially for women, age does become a consideration. Around my thirty-sixth birthday, it became a turning point for me – one where I knew I had to think seriously about timeframes and the future. I started to think about how neither me nor my partner had tried to have children before, and so there were still unknowns about the future. I'd think about how our age could possibly impact on the time it would take to conceive. And I also thought about our age when our child would be ten, twenty, thirty, or forty years old and what mine and my partner's lives would be like then.

Lastly, and most importantly for me, I found the person who I knew I wanted to raise children with and who would be a loving and caring father to our child. We've been together for five years and in that time, I have become more settled with my life and ready to bring children into the world.

These are just my thoughts and reasons and everybody will have a different experience when they feel ready to step into motherhood. Some people may not plan children, but it will happen anyway and often turn out beautifully. It might be that some of my reasons may have no bearing on other people reading this. And that's fine. We all have our own feelings, thoughts and backgrounds which will have an impact on the decisions that we make.

My Reflections

So, to conclude, there really is no quiz that you can take that will tell you that you are ready to start a family, and it is important to know that no one else can tell you when you are.

It is your decision; listen to what you are telling you.

There is no doubt lots to consider, as becoming a mum is difficult. There is certainly no denying that. Bringing another life into the world is massive and then being responsible for that child is life changing beyond words.

My final words on this subject is to look at your life through a holistic lens.

Emotionally, physically and practically: What is coming up? What can be influenced? What can't be changed? Can you work around this?

Never forget, there is always someone who is able to support you – reach out!

Website and helpful phone numbers:

NHS support resources: https://www.nhs.uk/pregnancy

MoneyHelper: A national charity offering money advice for parents – https://www.moneyhelper.org.uk/en/benefits/benefits-if-you-have-children/benefits-and-entitlements-to-claim-when-you-have-a-baby

National Childbirth Trust: A national charity for parents-to-be and new parents – https://www.nct.org.uk

Pregnancy Crisis Helpline: A national charity supporting birth trauma – https://pregnancycrisishelpline.org.uk/ 0800 368 9296

Family Lives: 0808 800 2222

Bout to begin...

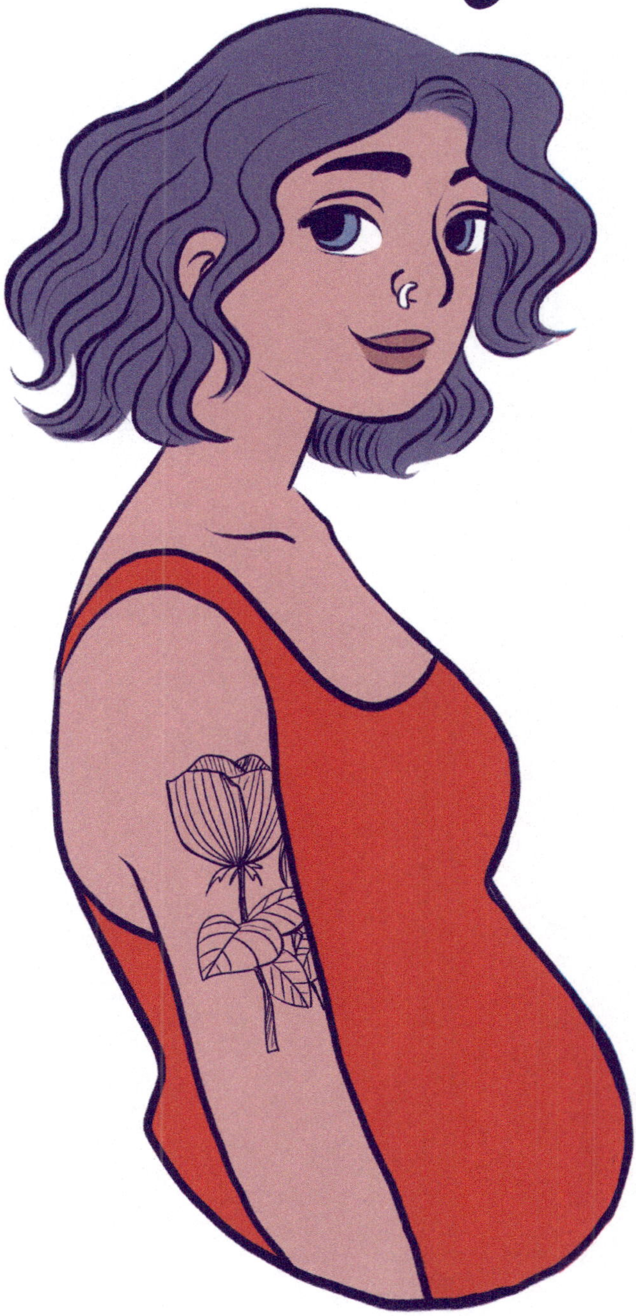

Somethin' is brewing – Becoming Pregnant

I am probably not the best person to write this, as I loved being pregnant with all three pregnancies. I felt it really suited me: no morning sickness, and even though I was VERY large for the second two, I just loved it. As already explained, none of my pregnancies were planned – I am not that organised! But I was ready, and as daft as it may sound, I felt that my body was also ready. Financially, we could have been better off but that certainly didn't impact the joy we both felt.

I have purposely chosen not to focus too much on other people's birth stories in this book. They are out there and everyone has their own story to tell. Birth, in my experience, is unique and always driven by the needs of the baby and mother in that moment, so I didn't feel it was appropriate to offer the personal stories of others here. But what this chapter will do is to capture pregnancy stories of both myself and others. For some, this stage can be crucial in preparing for the first year of motherhood.

This section is likely to be the longest section that I write. Each pregnancy and birth was very different and paints a clear picture of why I went on to do what I do now in my career.

My Pregnancies

My beautiful daughter

My first pregnancy came five years after having an ectopic pregnancy (which I go on to explain in more detail later in this book), but for those of you that don't know, ectopic pregnancies are very painful and the baby never survives. You are more likely to have an ectopic pregnancy after having one previously.

When I found out I was pregnant a second time I went into complete panic mode, worried the same thing would happen again.

It was Christmas Eve when I found out I was pregnant. Previously, I had always gone out on Christmas Eve with friends, but that year I had decided not to go as I was shattered and thought I would rest, especially as I was cooking lunch the next day. Steve went out and as I was sitting on my own, I started to think about how I had been feeling all week. I still don't know to this day what made me think about doing a pregnancy test, but I took myself off to the shop and came home and did a test.

Shocked when it came back positive, I rang Steve to come home and we went straight to A & E. I had already somehow convinced myself that it was going to happen again. The hospital was great and checked me over, giving me some reassurance to get through Christmas.

We had made the decision to tell the immediate family straight away, with it being Christmas. Everybody was so excited, and although Steve and I were, we were still shell-shocked and erring on the side of caution. I remember thinking next Christmas we could have a baby at home with us and what a different Christmas that would be. However, I was trying to not think too far ahead just in case the worst happened.

We were due to go away for New Year, so at the advice of the hospital team I went to see my GP who told me there was no reason why I shouldn't go away and thought it would be a good idea to rest. So, we went away, just Steve and I, which was great. It gave us a bit of space to talk about things and we both agreed we were excited but still very nervous. I was scared to go to the toilet just in case I noticed I was bleeding, but the week was lovely and was just what I needed.

As soon as the new year hit, I had a letter to attend an early scan due to the previous loss. We were so relieved to find out I was twelve weeks and all was fine, ectopic pregnancy was ruled out. I allowed myself to start to get excited – I was going to be a mum!

We didn't find out what we were having for any of our children and also didn't mention names to anyone. It wasn't even a conscious decision. Somebody asked why we didn't tell anyone; I think it was that we simply didn't know, especially for a girl – Steve and I had very different opinions on names!

Once I was reassured the pregnancy was all OK, it was a straightforward pregnancy. We went to birthing sessions that were held at the hospital as a couple, which focused on relaxation and mediation. I found the whole thing hilarious. At the time, it wasn't the sort of thing I did and certainly was not what Steve did. However, it was good for us to have conversations about the birth. We set a birth plan together and we were pretty much happy with anything, as long as the baby was healthy. Our only request was for Steve to cut the cord and tell me the sex of the baby.

I still laugh now about choosing our pram/ pushchair – it took forever to choose. I am not sure why; I wasn't the type to read magazines about pushchairs. I wasn't even too bothered about the most fashionable brand. I just remember wanting it to be extremely functional. I am a person who makes decisions quite promptly but when I have something in my mind I can be on a mission to find exactly what I have in my mind.

Here was my list of requirements at the time. I am pleased to say that the pram was perfect and I used it for all three children and still have it (just in case!!)

A Sprinkle of Light to Lead the Way - Choosing the right Pram

- *Is it a traditional pram? i.e. that a baby can lie down in*
- *Is it easy to fold up?*
- *Can it be used for long distance walks?*
- *Is it neutral in colour? (we didn't find out the gender of our babies)*
- *Can it be fitted into the car as a car seat?*

The final few weeks…

I worked up to four weeks before I had the baby and felt great. Everyone kept telling me that no babies come on the due date, so I was going with the flow and wasn't too focused on the due date of 13th August.

On 11th August, we went to a family BBQ and I remember feeling very tired so we didn't stay too long. During the night, I felt sick and was still very tired. When I told family members, they told me I probably had a stomach bug so I stayed in bed and tried to sleep it off. Later in the day, I started to bleed so called the maternity ward. I explained that I had a sickness bug and they asked me to call in because the bleeding was concerning. We walked in completely calm with no bag or anything, only to be told I was in the late stages of labour and definitely needed my bag – which luckily was in the car.

The birth was physically traumatic, resulting in a fourth degree tear after a forceps delivery. Our birth plan was kept to though and Steve cut the cord and told me the sex of the baby.

"Don't always believe that your first born will go past the due date."

Anyway, back to the birth. Even though it was a tough birth, I took one look at my daughter and love was instantly there! She was beautiful and perfect. I immediately forgot all that I had been through for the last six hours. We had told no one I had gone into hospital and so it was lovely to surprise everyone with the news.

Gracie Mai, weighing 7lbs 9. with her dad's long eyelashes and Mum's and Dad's very dark hair – I was completely smitten!

Gracie Mai, weighing 7lbs 9. with her dad's long eyelashes and Mum's and Dad's very dark hair – I was completely smitten!

The adorable giant

The day of Gracie Mai's first birthday party I knew I was pregnant again, my body was telling me. I absolutely was not trying for another and couldn't even remember having sex! I didn't know that you were likely to be more fertile in the first few months of having a baby. I was extremely apprehensive about having two under two; all I could think about was having a double pushchair! I had always thought I would have four years between the children, like my parents did with my sister and I. Steve was really happy and said having them close together is great as he is close in age to his brother.

The start of my pregnancy was all fine and was just like my first. I then went for my twenty-week scan and everything changed.

I instantly knew that there was a problem as there was so much silence and then those dreaded words: "I just need to go and get a consultant!" The doctor came and we were told to sit in the relative's room and the consultant would come and explain all.

Steve and I were told that they could see the baby's stomach developing inside the cord and that the baby may have Down's Syndrome. It was such a lot to process and lots of decisions needed to be made. We opted to have an amniocentesis to find out if the baby had Down's Syndrome. As you can imagine, this was a tough decision and many people judged us. We wanted to know either way to plan for our family's future. We had a one year old at home already who we needed to prepare for the forthcoming arrival; we also felt we needed to know so that the birth could be planned due to the stomach needing to be operated on at birth. We were told that if the baby had Down's Syndrome and with the stomach being where it was, it was likely the baby wouldn't survive more than a couple of hours.

I know I am writing this in a very matter-of-fact way. It is the only way I can. If I started to write about the anxiety, the fear and the trauma, I would never get through this chapter. When going through the situation, I could not give any emotion to it. My coping mechanism was to get on with it and stick with my head not the heart.

The three days waiting for the results were a blur for me as I went into my coping mode and kept myself busy. The results came back and the baby had none of the issues consultants were concerned about, but it was confirmed that the stomach was situated outside the body in the cord. I still to this day remember this phone call, even though it was good news. I cried once I heard the news and felt sick. The nurse confirmed with me that I had understood what she had said and offered reassurance. It made me realise how much I had been holding in, not wanting to face what may have laid ahead for us.

For the rest of the pregnancy, I was scanned every two weeks and I set a birth plan with the consultant. I felt empowered by this as I like to be in control of every situation as much as possible. Obviously, there was a lot out of my control in this case, which made it important for me to be able to control the bits I could.

It was made clear to me that at the birth the baby would be taken from me straight away and taken to Alder Hey in Liverpool. I seemed to focus on this information a lot; I now see that I was mentally preparing myself. At the birth, I would be immediately separated from my baby. I HAD to prepare myself. We were also told that he could be in Alder Hey for a while, so I spent a lot of my pregnancy planning this: Steve would need time from work, Gracie Mai would have to stay with grandparents, the dog would need sorting. The list went on.

I was distracted a lot of the time as Gracie Mai kept me busy, in a good way. I remember looking at her so many times when I was upset and she made me smile every time. I must admit that sometimes tiredness was on a different level. I had a one year old, I was getting heavily pregnant and the emotional stress of it all was exhausting at times. I was finding I wanted to rest more, and was becoming overwhelmed with all that was going on, crying when no one was around.

I was due to be induced on a Monday. It was decided that I would have a natural birth so I could follow the baby to Liverpool. My waters broke a week early at tea time. This sent me into panic as I felt 'THE PLAN' wasn't being followed. When I arrived at the hospital, they told me that the consultant was not in, but they assured me that they had the plan we had made and would keep to it. What I wasn't prepared for was how many people would be present in the room. It was really off-putting and I felt very exposed. I shared my feelings with the midwife, who closed the curtain so that only the people that needed to be with me were near me. After about four hours (I'm now not too sure how long exactly, to be honest!), I gave birth to a baby boy. Steve was able to cut the cord and tell me the sex, although at first his reaction was, "I don't know the sex but I know the baby is massive."

Baby was taken straight from me. I didn't get to see him but Steve did and said that he was huge. He was very swollen, particularly his stomach, and seemed to have no neck! Not painting a great picture, am I?! But he was so cuddly.

A few hours later, I was told our baby was in neonatal and I remember questioning why he was not on his way to Liverpool. No real answers were given at the time. All we were told was that they were struggling to stabilise him. What I wanted to know was what did that mean? How long would it be? What did they need to do to stabilise him? I was told to get some sleep and to call Steve to come back to the hospital (he had gone home to pack and settle our daughter).

When Steve came back, we were taken to see our baby boy. We were told that he was in a critical state as they could not stabilise his blood sugars. I was extremely tired and not really taking it all in. Steve was the same; there were periods of time when we just sat in silence. I think we were both overwhelmed with what had taken place and what was going to happen next – it was all unknown. It's the unknown and being out of control that I struggle with – yes, a control freak!

The hospital worked wonders and our baby was ready to go to Liverpool when he was fifteen hours old. We followed the ambulance all the way there. I was so happy I could do that. The natural birth and the damage was worth all the pain to be there as he went straight into theatre. We were offered a room within the Ronald McDonald house. Ronald McDonald houses are places for families to stay on-site at Alder Hey hospital. You have a room and a shared living room and kitchen space. This space was so special and important to us,

By this time, all the family knew that we had gone into hospital as they needed to look after Gracie Mai. As we hadn't known the sex of the baby beforehand or mentioned any names, it was a lovely surprise for them all once again. Even though it was a stressful time for all of us.

The operation was successful and our little boy's stomach was nice and neatly where it should be. The consultant stated that hopefully we would be going home within seventy-two hours. I held onto this. Then seventy-two hours passed, a week passed. Two, three, four weeks passed. Baby had lost a lot of weight and would not feed. At week two, we were told they suspected our son had a rare genetic disorder called Beckwith Wiedemann Syndrome, which ultimately meant he was born with adult-sized organs, hence why there was no room for his stomach. While at Alder Hey, we had genetic counselling. They went through all our family tree, asking about illnesses and long-standing health conditions. It was hard to think of answers at the time because I was so tired. We were supported throughout the diagnosis.

> *Lennon George, weighing 9 lbs 11 – another baby with lots of dark hair, a real little chunk.*

I remember being so upset as I had two children and neither were with me at Ronald McDonald House. Gracie Mai only came to stay with us on weekends and visited us during the week with other family members. She was only eighteen months herself and it was very difficult to explain to her what was going on. It was a challenging and traumatic few months that undoubtedly shaped me as a mum and the woman I am now.

A Sprinkle of Light to Lead the Way – Life on a special care baby unit

Having a baby in Special Care is an experience thankfully not many parents have to go through; it's still an experience I think about regularly. Looking back, here is what I would recommend to myself and others:

- *Ask any questions that you may have, no matter how trivial you think they are. If you don't understand the medical language, find someone you feel comfortable with and tell them you don't understand.*
- *Make sure your mental health and physical health is cared for. It's so easy for both professionals and yourself to forget you are still important.*
- *Don't feel guilty if you have to take time out, even if it's away from the hospital – it is important you take this time.*
- *If you have any fears, speak to the right people about them: consultants, family members, etc.*
- *If you have other children, try to spend time with them and explain to them what is going on (age appropriate).*

The perfect early bird

Fast forward three-and-a-bit years, I found myself pregnant again and I know a few were shocked that we went on to have another baby, due to the physical and emotional effects of the previous birth. Again, another unplanned pregnancy, but

I was happy although worried – understandably, given our previous experience. As Lennon got older, we were told that it was highly unlikely that another baby would have the same condition but I was still a little concerned. The pregnancy was classed as high risk due to my previous pregnancy so a plan was put into place. I was scanned early and was under a consultant throughout. I was scanned every two weeks, which I found reassuring.

I was so excited to tell Gracie Mai (who was now five years old) and Lennon (now four years) about the news. They were so thrilled and this made it all the more magical. The pregnancy was great, although tiring at times. I had two young children, was working part time as a support worker, was in my final year of my counselling degree and was on placement! I remember counselling at eight months' pregnant and my clients wanting reassurance that I wasn't going to go into labour during their session!

I shouldn't say this (don't judge me!) but I think this was my favourite pregnancy of them all. It didn't stop me from doing anything and I was in a job where everyone was excited for me. The kids were super enthusiastic and this made it really special. I had regular scans and was reassured all the way through.

I was sent for a scan of my vaginal area to assess the damage due to the previous two births being so physically traumatic. I was told that there was a lot of damage and that a caesarean was the best option. I was apprehensive due to not being able to drive for a while after a caesarean, but my family said that they would support the school run.

I had worked virtually right up to my due date with my older two, so this time I had planned to have a rest before and get ready for Christmas. My due date was 12/12/12 which was just a fab date to have!

I finished work a month before my due date with the plan being to get all the presents and Christmas preparation done. A great plan until my water broke literally two days into maternity leave. I went into the hospital and they checked me over and said that I wasn't yet in full labour. However, due to the amount of water I had lost and was still losing, they gave me a bed to stay in. I could feel labour coming on fast and we called a nurse in. She said that there were no spaces to take me down to the theatre so I had to wait until a space was free. My labour continued to be fast and again I called the nurse and told her I was sure the baby was coming. She checked me over and sure enough, she said the baby was indeed on its way. I gave birth within forty minutes with no pain relief. He was perfect and I was so happy. Steve again cut the cord and told me it was a baby boy.

Dylan James, weighing 7 lbs 4, our smallest baby, with the smoothest olive skin and beautiful dark hair.

We went home within twelve hours and my other two adored him.

Other than him being in hospital when he was four weeks old for his first Christmas (he had bronchitis and was in for a week, but soon recovered), it was a lovely birth. Having said that, I will say more about the complications when he was back in hospital in the next section.

Dylan James, weighing 7 lbs 4, our smallest baby, with the smoothest olive skin and beautiful dark hair.

"Try to get as much rest as possible leading up to your due date. I know you will want to get everything done and make everything perfect for your little one, but rest /self-care really is the most important. Try to find a balance that works for you."

OK, so now you know all about my pregnancies and early days of my three beautiful children, take a read of others' experiences.

The Mental Health Impact – Danielle's story

The day my (then) husband and I found out we were expecting our first child, it was pure joy and happiness from both sides. Little did we expect such trauma to follow.

I had some physical problems throughout the pregnancy, such as bad sickness all the way through and pre-eclampsia at the end. However, my mental health especially was affected from about two months pregnant.

"After a couple of months of being pregnant, my mental health deteriorated. I was very anxious and depressed and had some dark thoughts."

I got allocated a midwife from the mental health/safeguarding team after the midwife at my initial appointment referred me because of my mental health issues (Obsessive Compulsive Disorder, Borderline Personality Disorder and Depressive and anxiety disorder). She said I would need extra support as pregnancy can make mental health issues worse, and she was right in my case.

After a couple of months of being pregnant, my mental health deteriorated. I was very anxious and depressed and had some dark thoughts. My relationship was strained and my ex-husband was becoming nasty with me because he didn't understand mental health issues.

I became close to my midwife and she was my biggest support. I saw her once or twice a week and she knew how much I was struggling. As time went on, I became worse and also psychotic at times – I was a risk to myself. My midwife got concerned and referred me to social services for extra support for when the baby was here and got me a family support worker involved too.

The social worker wasn't very nice or supportive, and the way she treated me still affects me today. I still think about it almost six years later. I was about twenty-eight weeks pregnant when she came to our house and sat me and my ex-partner down and said that the baby would be taken from us at birth because of my mental health. It was a bit of a blur. I couldn't stop the tears and was having a bad panic attack. My life was over. The social worker continued to say that they would take our baby at birth then take us to court for parental responsibility.

However, the thought of being a mum kept me going. I knew things would get better once the baby was here, once my hormones had calmed down and I could go back on the medication I had to stop taking, which had worked well for me when I was on them. I loved our baby so much and he was keeping me alive. We had some meetings and a few more appointments. After fighting some more, they were considering giving us a chance and putting our baby on a child protection plan and giving us a parenting assessment.

At thirty-nine weeks pregnant it was time for my c-section, and we still didn't know whether we would be allowed to take our baby home. I was numb. I can't remember much because I think I blocked the memories out.

We had a meeting booked with the professionals involved after he was born. Everybody came into the side room and sat on a chair in a circle. We were praying for the right outcome. I couldn't bear it and was holding my baby son to my

> We all discussed our baby and, much to our huge relief, they were going to give us a chance.

chest. How could I possibly let him go? I was so worried about bonding with him in case he was taken but already the love was unconditional. We all discussed our baby and, much to our huge relief, they were going to give us a chance.

However, for the first three months I had to be supervised with him twenty-four hours a day and he would be put on a child protection plan while they completed parenting assessments. My family and my ex-husband's family made a rota, ensuring that someone was with me at all times. It was frustrating but at least I had my baby. My mental health started to improve and social services did their assessment and closed the case. We also got an apology from the social worker's manager after everything because of how badly we were treated.

My pregnancy – Nic's story

My pregnancy was really unusual. When my pregnancy began, my husband was sectioned in a mental health ward.

He had been unwell with undiagnosed bipolar for some weeks before that. It had finally come to a head and they decided to keep him in if he tried to leave. He was kept on the section for a month, and it was during a planned visitation home that one thing led to another and two weeks later, at home alone, I did a test and discovered I was pregnant.

It was hard to begin with, not because of the pregnancy itself, but because of people's

> At our twelve-week scan I couldn't actually believe that the little bean on the screen was mine and growing inside me. It all felt so surreal.

reaction to it. J's section hadn't gone unnoticed by both of our families, and my parents in particular were disappointed. I knew that whatever I was going through though, we'd come out of it stronger, and our baby would be so loved. In the first few weeks I was incredibly lucky and had zero symptoms: no sickness, no tenderness, nothing. This made me question whether I was actually pregnant! I must have done about twenty pregnancy tests just to make sure. At our twelve-week scan I couldn't actually believe that the little bean on the screen was mine and growing inside me. It all felt so surreal, and that's when pregnancy hit me. I suffered with Symphysis Pubis Dysfunction (SPD) for fifteen weeks. SPD is a collection of uncomfortable symptoms caused by a stiffness of your pelvic joints or the joints moving unevenly at either the back or front of your pelvis. This usually resolves after you have given birth. There are a number of treatments to try and limit the symptoms, and one of those I used was a bump band that adds extra support to your growing tummy. This also added a wonderful waddle just trying to move around the house! At twenty weeks we went for our anomaly scan and discovered we were having a baby girl! We began getting together lots of baby clothes and the larger items after the scan, as we were a bit more into the clear.

Just after the scan we moved into a new home, which was stressful but we luckily had a lot of support at the time and I was banned from the heavy lifting. Most of my day was spent sitting in the moving van making sure no one damaged it – mainly because I couldn't get back in the van more than once so I was stuck there!

I started getting these weird feelings, like my bladder would twitch, and it took me a few days to realise that it was actually me feeling baby movements for the first time! As the baby got bigger I loved feeling it moving and I could watch the arms and legs jutting out and sweeping around. It's the one thing I really miss about pregnancy. When I got to thirty-two weeks, I began my maternity leave. I was working in a travel money bureau and spent up to twelve hours a day in a Perspex box – even prisoners get more room than we did in there! It was summer 2012 and it was ridiculously hot! My feet often didn't look like feet anymore because they were so swollen! I spent most of my maternity leave before birth with my feet elevated and watching Four in a bed on TV, scarfing down jacket potatoes with lots of cheese. I'm surprised baby didn't come out looking like a potato!

At thirty-six weeks my mum came to visit while we went for a growth scan to make sure the baby wasn't too big. We had just decided on the baby's name as Ellie the night before. When we were at the hospital, Mum asked them to check the baby's gender. She just had a feeling, and it's a good job she asked as they revealed that actually our baby had a scrotum so definitely wasn't a girl! Wow, it was a shock. A happy shock. Ringing everyone to tell them the news was just hilarious, and I kept randomly bursting into laughter for the next few days. Back to the drawing board on names! I had a friend who was three months behind me and pregnant with a girl, so thankfully all of the girls' items went to her for her baby.

My due date came and went with no sign. I had a 'Stretch and Sweep', which is a small medical procedure to try and bring on labour, and he still refused to come out. So at forty weeks and five days I was admitted to hospital to be induced. It was hot, and I was very uncomfortable. Five days after my due date, the consultant had agreed to go ahead with induction. I was given the pessary at 5 p.m., and by 7 p.m. I was getting regular contractions. At 9 p.m., my husband was sent home. Ward visiting hours were over. I was in so much pain! I was perched on the edge of the bed because I couldn't sit back, the pressure was too much. I tried people watching out of the window, and hooking up my TENS machine (which did nothing more than mildly distract me when I zapped myself). I buzzed the midwife because I couldn't take it anymore. She came and said I could have some paracetamol in an hour. I felt like throwing her out of the window at this point, and then telling her she could only have paracetamol! The lady in the bed next to me was being induced at the same time as I was. She admitted she was jealous – mine had worked and hers hadn't.

When the midwife came back with the paracetamol, she told me to get ready for the doctor to come and examine me – FINALLY! I admit, it took me about fifteen minutes to get on the bed because of the pressure and how awkward it was to undress, but finally I was there! And the lovely doctor came in and began his examination – I held my breath, hoping all this pain was worth it. "Well," he said, "you're about four centimetres. Let's get you down to the labour ward." Cue me bursting into tears and declaring my undying love for him. I had the go-ahead. I was in labour! Not long after I had given birth and I had this gorgeous baby boy in my arms. He was all mine, cooked to perfection.

"I had this gorgeous baby boy in my arms. He was all mine, cooked to perfection."

Spoonful of Love from Nic

"Remember that the hospital does not always get the gender correct at the scan. Try not to get too carried away buying gender-specific items before the birth. There have been a few surprises!"

Expecting the Unexpected – Kirsten's story

When I was younger, I did a lot of babysitting, saw a lot of different pregnancies, and heard many different birth stories. Never the same one twice. And this rang true for my own pregnancies. Two very different children and two very different experiences of pregnancy.

> Two very different children and two very different experiences of pregnancy.

The first time round, I couldn't stop eating. Anything apart from chicken, that is. I remember my husband getting a take out and I had to open all the doors and windows to get rid of the smell. Normally, I love chicken, but everything about it back then was revolting.

The second time, most food was repulsive. Unless it was covered in maple syrup. "It's not a craving – it's perfectly normal! Look!" I said to my other half, showing him random photos I'd found in the depths of the internet. Pizza, avocado, chips and other tasty delights drizzled with the stuff.

With my first, I was working teaching English to adults a few days a week and could rest in between. I ballooned up quickly (turned out to be pre-eclampsia in the end but that's another much longer story!) What struck me, though, was that pregnancy seemed to give everyone a green light to comment on what I was eating and how I looked. "Isn't your bump big!" "You look like you're eating well!" It made me feel self-conscious next to more petite pregnant friends who got comments such as, "Aw, look at your neat bump!", "Oh you've got that pregnancy glow!", "You're hardly showing at all!" I don't normally take comments to heart, but hormones and emotions were heightened and often I'd end up feeling like a prize heifer being judged.

By the time I was pregnant with my second son, my skin was much thicker and I cared less about what others thought. And besides, I was too busy running around after my eighteen-month-old to have the luxury of time to worry about what other people did or didn't think of my bump.

> If I'd had a rigid birthing plan, I don't think I would have mentally recovered as quickly.

I remember being asked about birthing plans. First time around, I remember a pregnant friend saying, "As long as everyone is happy and healthy, if the baby is born out of my elbow, I don't care!" So I listened to the options and scribbled a rough draft, but realised that nothing was set in stone. This turned out to be a huge positive. The birth was six weeks early and didn't go quite as planned. If I'd had a rigid birthing plan, I don't think I would have mentally recovered as quickly. The second time round, though, I had a little cry as the consultant said "No way" to the "As natural as possible" birthing centre birth I'd imagined. It turned out to be the right call, though (preeclampsia struck again!), and as my husband pointed out, safely and healthily is best. Both births were c-sections and this was the best option for me.

Spoonful of Love from Kirsten

"If I've learned anything, it's that it's good to question and get checked if something doesn't feel right and to listen to our bodies. Pregnancies and births come in all shapes and sizes. There is no one rule that fits all."

Reflections

Continuing with what Kirsten has just said – there really is no one rule fits all.

You will have read from my varying pregnancies and immediate days after, no one would have expected how each one went.

If you're reading this book and are still considering having children, I do hope that this chapter hasn't put you off! I look at each one of my pregnancies now with fond memories, and even though some situations were extremely difficult at the time, it has defined me as a mum and a woman.

If you have had children and are reading this book, I would love to hear how your pregnancy has defined you as a mum.

Pregnancy is an important stage on the mothering journey. No, it is not an illness, but a mum should be cared for. The journey ahead is a long and winding road.

Websites and helpful phone numbers:

NHS advice and guidance: https://www.nhs.uk/pregnancy

Pregnancy Crisis Helpline: A national charity supporting birth trauma – https://pregnancycrisishelpline.org.uk/ 0800 368 9296

PANDAS: A national charity supporting Post Natal Depression – https://pandasfoundation.org.uk

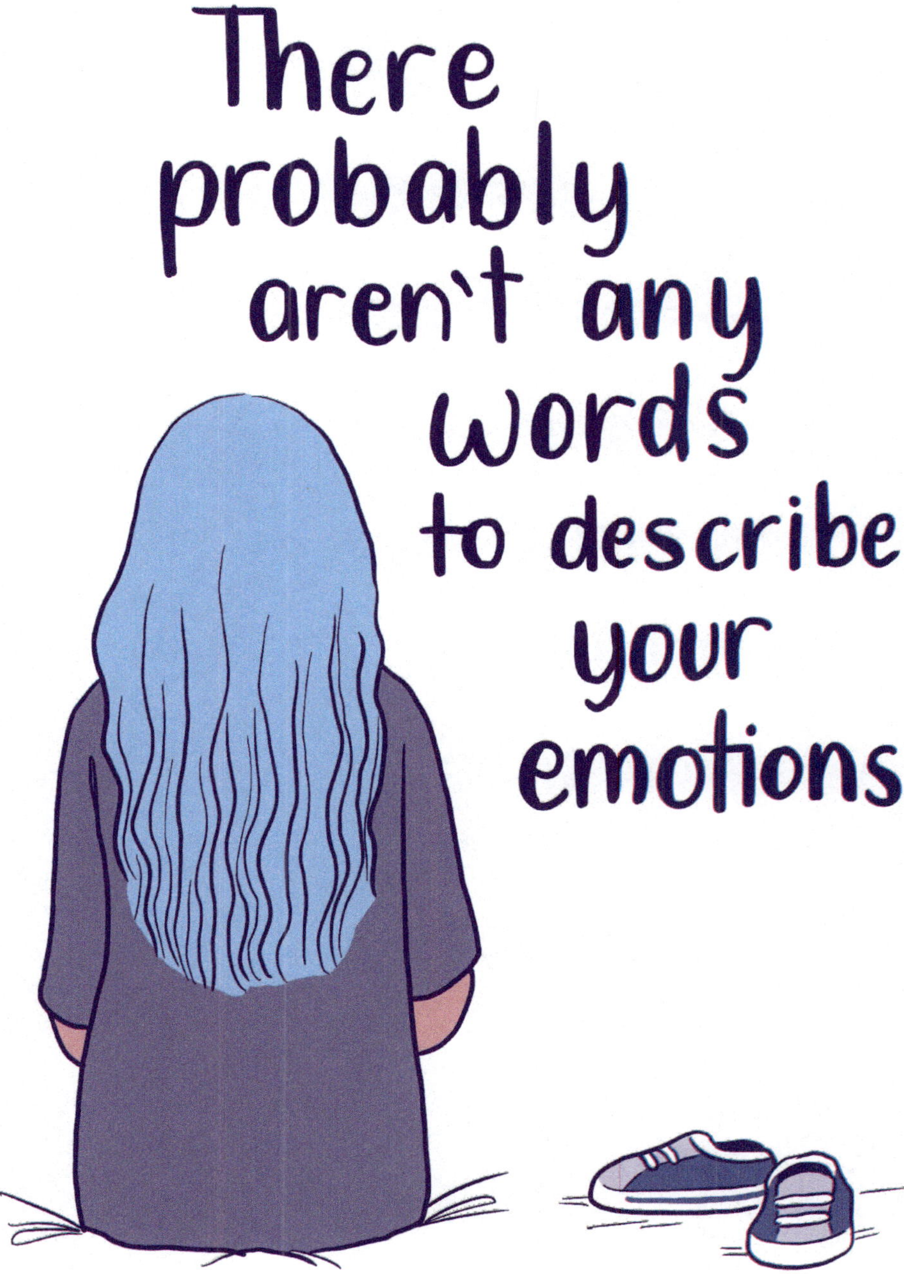
There probably aren't any words to describe your emotions

There probably aren't words to describe your emotions - Experience of infant loss

I really didn't know where this section should sit in this book, but for me this chapter sits here as it follows my life journey.

Despite the ups and downs of the birth process, most mothers would not swap it for the world because of what they have because of it. However, not everyone is so lucky. Infant loss and child loss is unfortunately something that many have experienced.

This chapter focuses on that harrowing subject of infant loss and child loss, a difficult topic for many to read but to me a crucial area to cover. As a counsellor, my specialist area is infant loss and I have worked with many individuals who have experienced loss. Many who feel extremely lonely, isolated and lost in grief.

I have experienced an ectopic pregnancy, miscarriage and (I haven't told many people this) also a termination. Regarding the termination, I have battled with myself whether I should include it in the book but feel it is right to do so.

I pride myself on being honest with everyone that I come into contact with – and this book is no different. Some people may not feel that writing about a termination in this section is the right place to do so, and I absolutely accept that, but for others, I know this is how they feel about it. Many women experience a real internal struggle. It is a baby loss and can have a deep emotional impact. I have seen this first hand.

My first loss

Firstly, focusing on my ectopic pregnancy, which I have mentioned earlier in this book. I was only twenty-three years old when I found out I was pregnant – there is a bit of a backstory to this so please bear with me!

At twenty-three, I was a project manager in retail, working with a team to get large clothing stores open, working thirteen-plus hours a day. I enjoyed it; the buzz of getting the stores open on time as well as the team approach to the achievement was a real high for me.

I had just finished opening a store and had two days off before flying out to Cuba with Steve. I was absolutely exhausted, but the thought of a nice holiday was keeping me going. Then, just like that, everything changed. I was talking to my neighbour in the garden when I collapsed. I felt awful, completely weak. I spoke to both my mum and Steve, who convinced me to go to see the GP and get checked out before the holiday. So off I went and explained that I thought it was exhaustion due to my job. The GP asked me to do a pregnancy test as a precaution. I explained that this wasn't needed as I was on the pill and always very careful. The test came back positive; I could not believe it! The GP explained that it was likely all was fine, that like I said I was just tired, but wanted me to cancel the holiday just in case, as being on a twelve-hour flight could put both unborn baby and myself in a dangerous position until things calmed down.

To this day, I remember walking out of the surgery and telling my mum, thinking that this couldn't be happening: I don't want to be a mum, I am not ready, I want to go on holiday. My mum was so pleased and excited. I was the opposite but didn't say anything. I went home and, as I saw it at the time, broke the 'bad' news to Steve. We did cancel the holiday and that night I don't remember speaking much about it; in fact, I was probably so shocked that I didn't.

The next day I woke up with the worst pain I have ever experienced – still to this day, I have not experienced pain like it. We called the GP who told me to go in the bath as it was likely I was miscarrying. During the night, I was still in pain and in the morning the pain was excruciating, and I was bleeding very heavily. We called the GP again and they explained that it was still likely to be a miscarriage, but due to the bleeding, they called an ambulance to come and collect me to take me to A & E. Once in A & E, I waited a long time to be seen. The pain was becoming more and more intense. Eventually, I was seen by a doctor who then asked me to go to maternity to be scanned. After lots of coming and going, I was eventually told that I was having an ectopic pregnancy. I had no idea what this meant medically but I did know that just a few weeks earlier The Countess of Wessex had suffered an Ectopic Pregnancy and it stated on the news that she was very close to death and the air ambulance was crucial to her survival. So, I did ask if I was likely to die! Looking back, I know this sounds so dramatic but I knew no other person who had had the same experience and no one was explaining anything to me. It was eventually explained that I was not at risk and was now in the best place and would be taken to theatre, but there was no way that the baby would survive.

I was prepped for theatre twice and got half way down the corridor, but due to a busy theatre, I was sent back down to the ward. On the third attempt, I was taken to the theatre but before they started to operate, my Fallopian tube ruptured, causing me to also have my right tube removed.

After the operation, a consultant came and explained all that had happened to me. It was explained that with now only having one tube, it could reduce my chances of becoming a mum.

So within thirty-six hours, I had gone from being a project manager, very carefree, with lots to look forward to, due to go to Cuba, to being in the hospital, being told I had lost my baby and my chances of having another baby may be reduced.

“Listen to your body, my body was telling me I was exhausted and something was wrong, but I chose not to listen.”

Due to the operation, I had to take time off work – which was unheard of for me. However, it gave me a chance to reflect and review my priorities. While I was on leave, redundancies came up at work as part of a restructure and I applied. For the first time, I was starting to think about being a parent, and the possibility of not being able to have children was on my mind. Work didn't want me to leave and persuaded me not to go – they offered me quite a sizable pay rise. However, I declined. I was angry with them; I resented how hard I had worked for them. I was constantly tired and hadn't realised I was pregnant and now I faced the possibility of not being able to have children. I wanted someone to blame and they were my target.

A couple of weeks later, I started to experience nightmares and struggled to get to sleep. I mentioned them to the GP at my post-op check-up and she said that it was the anxiety after what had happened. I was shocked. Anxiety was not something I had, surely. That just wasn't me.

I look back now and think that was exactly what it was. I overcame this anxiety because I never returned to the hustle and bustle of my job. Instead, I was fortunate that I went into a job that was not pressured and didn't have long hours. From there, I started to train as a counsellor. It was while training as a counsellor I learnt about trauma, both physical and emotional, and I began to understand that my body was still suffering trauma. Still to this day, when I get stressed, I have a pain in my side where my tube was removed. As the saying goes, "the body remembers." I don't know if any of you can relate to this kind of trauma. Over the last twelve years as a counsellor I have met many women who have

> *I will always remember this loss, a loss of a baby, a loss of part of me, the loss of a job.*

also had an ectopic pregnancy and we have spoken about the physical trauma that takes place in the aftermath of such a painful loss.

Just for your information, I was told that it was the contraception pill that I was on that had caused the ectopic pregnancy, so I had to look at a more suitable contraception for future use.

I will always remember this loss, a loss of a baby, a loss of part of me, the loss of a job.

"Never minimise the sense of loss an ectopic pregnancy can bring."

A very different kind of loss

As you will have gathered, I did go on to have children. I was told that my left tube was still very healthy and there should be no reason why I couldn't have children.

At one stage, I had two children under two, which was not easy, especially with Lennon being ill. It took me a long time to readjust to being a mum of two and to come to terms with the trauma of what had happened with Lennon in the early months. With having a natural birth, my body was also not the best, with Lennon being such a big baby, I had a lot of interior problems, which I will explore later in this book.

Things were starting to settle down and the four of us were getting into a nice routine. When Lennon was eight months, I felt quite unwell and tired all the time. I started to consider that I may be pregnant and for a couple of days I put off doing a test as I didn't want to face the answer. I eventually did the test and unbelievably it was positive. I honestly can't remember ever even having sex to conceive. I was devastated. I knew financially that we would struggle – I was only working part time at the time as I had taken time out to be with the two children and be with Lennon with him being unwell. However, money is money and we knew that we would cope financially. What I couldn't guarantee was how I would have coped. Although never diagnosed, I look back and would say I was suffering from postnatal depression – mildly, but definitely post trauma after what had taken place over the previous twelve months. I simply could not have imagined having another child.

Steve and I discussed our options at length and it was decided that terminating the pregnancy was best for the family. Even writing this, I fear judgement, but all

I can say is that it was not a decision that I took lightly. However, to this day, it's not a decision that I regret.

On the day of the termination itself, I was so upset, filled with a range of emotions. Frightened, guilty, overwhelmed, etc. The clinic itself was great and I was surprised at how busy it was and how fast everything took place.

As I write this, there are only five people that know about this. Writing this, I am exploring why I have not told more people. I know the answer – fear of judgement, and that it is not something that I am proud of. However, what I would say is that I am proud that we are in a country where the right to choose is available and that support is available for women to explore the options that are available for them.

"Making the decision to terminate a pregnancy is never an easy one for anyone. Get support from people/professionals who you know will support you through such a difficult time."

A painful loss that was the seed to something better

There is yet another long and complicated back story to this loss – bear with me!

My children were now getting older but all under 12. I was on the contraception pill when I started to bleed a lot in between periods and was getting pain from the vagina area at periods throughout the months. I was checked out by the GP who referred me to a gynaecological consultant. I was tested for being pregnant by the GP before I went to see the consultant and this came back negative. Further tests were carried out by the consultant to eliminate any cancers being the cause – this was a little alarming but I was reassured that it was more to rule out than anything else.

Over the Christmas break, I was waiting to go back for more tests in the new year. I was still bleeding, and I was noticing that it was becoming progressively heavier, but then some days I was just spotting. It was all very random and I had no idea each day what would take place. As we went into the new year, the bleeding started to get heavier and heavier but with no real pain. In my mind, I kept thinking everything was going to be OK because I had my appointment with the consultant coming up and would just explain everything to her.

Then one Friday night, I went to the toilet and was surprised at the flood of blood. I also had a mild stomach cramp. I don't really know why I didn't call the doctor at this stage, but I kept thinking it was only two more weeks until my appointment. The pain and the bleeding settled and the next day was a bit better – until the evening. Again, I felt like I needed the toilet and had a mild stomach pain. I went to the toilet and could see that I was bleeding heavily. This time it didn't stop, and without going into graphic detail, I was unable to leave the bathroom. The pain was becoming more and more extreme, like very sharp stomach cramps. I called Steve in and it was decided it was best for him to take the children out to my sister as we were due to go to my sister's for tea anyway.

Once the family left, I managed to get myself upstairs and called 111. As soon as Steve had told my sister what was happening, she came to see me at home and Steve stayed with the kids at her house.

After a long wait (surprise, surprise), I went through a series of questions with 111 and they decided, due to the blood loss, that I needed an ambulance. The ambulance came and took me and my sister to A & E. By this point, I had extreme stomach cramps and was bleeding very heavily. I was taken into a side room and blood was everywhere, so much so that the nurse had to pop in every ten minutes or so to mop up. However, I still hadn't seen anyone to talk to about what was going on. Then after about an hour, it was very clear that I was experiencing a miscarriage due to what was passing. Without being too graphic, it was clear what was taking place. We called a nurse in, who agreed with our assessment and got me to do a pregnancy test (Which to be honest, I wasn't sure why; surely it was going to be negative now?). They also took samples of what I was passing to be analysed. Once it was clear what was taking place, I was moved to the Gynaecology ward and medics assisted me to pass the rest of the foetus. It was extremely painful because no pain relief had kicked in as I had only just been offered it.

I stayed in overnight as the medics wanted to monitor me due to the amount of blood that I had lost. I was given a side room on the ward and there was a lovely nurse that kept popping in to see me during the night. I remember feeling grubby as I hadn't showered or bathed and also felt cold as I had gone in with limited layers and no socks.

The next morning, a consultant came in and said she would scan me but didn't really explain why. I had an internal scan and the consultant said to me, "It's all gone now so you can go home." I was so struck by how cold her manner was. No empathy and no compassion. She then failed to tell anyone else that I could go home, so I sat there waiting for ages until a nurse noticed I was all dressed and asked, "Are you allowed to go home now?" I answered yes and she said she would get my paperwork processed and get a lift arranged.

I was SO angry about this. Even writing this now, I feel angry about it. When I went into the hospital the night before, I didn't know I was pregnant. However, I could have known, and if I had, I would have been absolutely devastated leaving the hospital the way that I did. Even so, it was traumatic to lose a baby, having just been told I was around fourteen weeks pregnant. I felt very alone, and completely bewildered as to what had gone on.

I felt numb for quite a long time after, but focused on my work and the other children to get me through. A few months later, I decided to blog about my experience and was shocked to receive so many messages from people locally who had gone through very similar experiences. So, I decided to do something about it and set up what is now known as our Cherry Blossom project that is part of our charity, offering peer support and counselling for women who have experienced infant loss. A project that has supported hundreds of women since my loss in 2017. Something that I am very proud of.

A Sprinkle of Light to lead the way – Healing from loss

Loss and trauma can impact you both physically and emotionally and it's vital you offer yourself self-care to recover. After loss, it's important that:

- *You don't compare your loss with others; grief is personal.*

  You speak to others to process your thoughts when YOU feel ready to do so.
- *You do what is right for you at the time – grief is a journey.*

  You also need self-care and to look after yourself following the physical trauma.
- *As mentioned previously, it is perfectly acceptable to grieve a loss through termination – don't let anyone tell you different.*

These are my experiences and I am thankful for the support that I have had along the way, from health professionals, friends, family and third sector organisations. It has been a holistic approach.

Everyone who has experienced infant loss has their own story and each of their losses is unique and should not be judged or compared.

Thank you to each mum who has shared their experiences here:

A difficult loss – Violet's story

Writing this is hard. I have wanted to talk about my loss from day one, but when I compare it to others, I feel like a fraud.

I guess I should start back when I first knew. I woke from a vivid dream, a nightmare – you know the type, the ones where you suddenly wake up, believing for a second that it's real, sitting up, then realising it's just a dream and lying back down again. I dreamt I was in a hospital bed, a baby in a crib next to me. I begged the midwife to let me have my baby – not the one lying there, which I didn't even glance at, but the other, the one I hadn't seen, whisked away as soon as it was born. I didn't even know if it was male or female. Then I was suddenly standing in a hospital corridor, my husband in the doorway to the car park behind me, holding a baby in a car seat. I had my back to them, and I was trying to get back through the other door, to the ward. I was begging the nurse to give me my baby, screaming and crying. She said, "You have one, be happy with that," and closed the door. I woke in tears, believing there had been twins and that for some unexplained reason, one had been taken, and could never come home.

> You have one, be happy with that.

When I realised it was just a dream, I also realised I might be pregnant – not planned, not really affordable or particularly wanted. I went to a midwife, who looked at dates. Four weeks later I went for a scan. My husband had trouble parking, so they let me wait, but then said I'd have to go in. I prayed he'd park in time to join me. They did the scan before he got there – there it was, a baby, healthy and growing. Then she showed me, next to it, a much smaller foetus, undeveloped, no heartbeat, and said the words, "I'm very sorry, but as you can see, there was a twin which unfortunately hasn't survived." She asked if I was OK. I said I was. I said I knew; I told her in brief about my dream. She looked surprised and then told me the twin had stopped developing at roughly eight weeks. At that point, someone appeared to say my husband was there, and to check if it was the right room and could he come in. The sonographer asked if I wanted to tell him or if she should. I asked her to. He didn't really react. When the scan was over, we were asked if we wanted a photo – we both said yes. My husband took it. We were asked to go and wait in the waiting room as I had said I wanted the test for Down's Syndrome.

The waiting room was crowded. We sat down in the only place with two seats left together. I looked at the photo – my beautiful baby ... no twin! I was shocked and upset; the one chance to have a lasting memory of that twin and they hadn't given it to me, they hadn't even asked, just cut the dead baby out. I looked around, wanting to get another photo, and saw signs saying, 'Please make sure you are happy with your scan photos before leaving the room as scans cannot be repeated'. Then I looked straight in front of me – we were sitting directly in front of a board with information on multiple births, twins and more, TAMBA. I wanted to cry but no tears would come.

I wanted to cry but no tears would come.

We were called by a nurse to go into a room where she explained that because of the twin, they couldn't do the blood tests – the DNA would potentially give an incorrect result. I was asked if I wanted to talk to anyone about the twin. By that point, I was just in shock, so I shook my head. I couldn't speak, and my husband said no, we were fine. We went home.

I remember telling people – I wanted people to know it had been twins. For me, they had to know that there had been two babies. My husband told his family but not others. I told everyone. I remember the reactions: a very good but very tactless friend told me, "Yes, it's sad, but when you think about it it's probably for the best. You struggle with one baby so you wouldn't cope with two." Another good friend who isn't particularly fond of kids and definitely not religious lit a candle for my baby and sent me a photo of it burning. It was so comforting to have it recognised in that way. I was distraught; I cried every night after my children went to bed and my husband had gone to work. I guess at this point I should explain that my husband works nights, I have two older boys (older, but only four and two at that point), I use a crutch to walk, and had had postnatal depression fairly severely twice – perhaps now you agree with the first friend? In my head, I tried to convince myself that was logical, it was how I should feel. But I didn't. I was distraught. My baby was dead. I needed to know if it was just a thing that my body would reabsorb, or a baby with a soul feeling the love in heaven I could never give on earth. My minister spoke to me. She was reassuring but didn't give false hope. She said we couldn't know for sure, but that we could hope it was with God and pray.

Time passed. At the next appointment with my community midwife, I told her it had been twins and then she checked the notes to confirm that. She asked if I wanted to hear my baby's heartbeat. I did. It took her a while to find it. I think she could see I was starting to panic. She tried to reassure me; she said it didn't normally take that long, but the noise I could hear was the baby's blood flow, so it was definitely there and the reason it was taking so long is that every time she found it, it moved, so she knew there was a heartbeat. I hadn't realised how much I was panicking until she finally found it and I felt the relief wash over me.

> The twin wasn't really mentioned after that in the hospital, they simply confirmed it had vanished by the twenty-week scan.

The twin wasn't really mentioned after that in the hospital, they simply confirmed it had vanished by the twenty-week scan. I had regular appointments for gestational diabetes but the team involved in that side of things never mentioned it at all.

My minister had promised me that when my son is baptised, we can include the twin in the ceremony – I don't know how, but I'm glad, although I know it will probably have me in tears and confuse a lot of those attending. She was lovely; no body, no burial, but she organised a private 'funeral'. She did an order of service, just herself, me, my husband and our boys, at the church. It was simple, but perfect. My husband told me he hadn't realised how much he needed it until he attended – until that point it hadn't felt real to him. I guess men really do feel things differently. The minister asked if we knew if it was a boy or girl, or if we had a name. My husband said no. I knew what I was having with my first two... with this one, I didn't. I kept veering from one to the other. This was a non-identical twin, so in my mind the reason I couldn't decide is because there was one of each. We had to wait for the birth to see which had survived.

> There is nothing on his birth certificate to state he ever had a twin.

When our son was born, the midwives in the birth suite and nurses on postnatal knew nothing about the twin, or didn't mention it. His health visitor didn't know until I told her. There is nothing on his birth certificate to state he ever had a twin.

I took a photo of the pages of my notes that mentioned it. I should have checked at the time, but I wasn't thinking – now I can see they are blurred. I needed people to know the twin existed, so I included them in the birth announcement. My mum was surprised – she had forgotten he was a twin, and wondered if it would surprise others.

Each of my children has a stamp used on their birth announcement. For my son, I chose a rabbit looking up, but I needed something for the twin too. I chose a butterfly. The twin also needed its own words in the announcement. I spent hours trawling the internet, looking for how to word it. In the end, I went with a simple quote, which I had already had made into a Christmas ornament. The final announcement had the rabbit looking up at a cut out butterfly swooping down. Inside was my son's birth announcement. On the inside cover was his twin's stamp, a beautiful sparkling butterfly, and the quote: "Not all twins walk side by side, sometimes one has wings to fly." I didn't need to find more words than that; it was enough to tell people and to invite them to acknowledge it.

When we went home, the tears started again. When I looked down at him, so small in my arm, my other arm hanging loosely by my side: space for another baby; space on his playmat; space in his basket.

OK, he's grown, he fills those spaces now, but the gaping hole in my heart is still there. I love him. I grieve for his twin. I feel guilty that he isn't enough. I feel guilty that people with one baby who miscarry lose everything and carry on somehow and I make a fuss about a lost twin when I have a beautiful healthy baby. I didn't have to go through a physical miscarriage – my body reabsorbed the twin. I feel so unbearably sad. I feel my heart is broken. I look at him, and just sometimes I see a shadow. I have to remember – I'm not sure how yet – but that baby is there, with me, part of me forever, and I need its brother to know too. I need him to know he is enough, he is loved, but that he had a twin whom I will always love and miss too.

When I count to where eight weeks in the pregnancy was, it's this week, baby loss awareness week, and I really do believe we need to talk about it. I've seen people say it in various ways, and here's mine – I'm a mum of four; three boys and one angel. I'll never forget.

A misunderstood loss – Francis' Story

I want to share my story of medical termination in 2010. A heart-aching decision which I still carry around with me today. I wanted to share as it's a story rarely told and a subject where women are faced with shame and feelings of judgement from others.

I found out I was pregnant at two weeks, the morning-after pill from the pharmacist hadn't worked two weeks before. I was a mum to two young children.

I went back to the same pharmacist and she led me to the same quiet room for a chat. She was kind and a good listener; she supported me to find out my next options. I knew what I was considering and she was there as I rang a local clinic for an appointment. She did not rush me and I felt safer with her than going into the doctors.

I had to wait for a phone call back. The next day a lady from the clinic rang and spoke to me, explaining exactly what happened during the process. I was sure this is what I wanted although I felt sad at the decision. She explained what happens at the two appointments and the aftercare. I booked an appointment for their earliest slot, which was two weeks later.

At four weeks pregnant I went along to the first appointment at the clinic. I felt sad, scared, nervous, and most of all terrified of having a pregnancy scan, an internal scan which is a probe to detect a gestational sac with an embryo. The first signs of a heartbeat is at about six weeks of pregnancy. At this appointment I needed to complete paperwork for consent. None of this information was shared with my doctors and it felt very private.

The clinic was in a discreet setting in South Manchester and outside it simply said the building name with a sign saying private clinic. (Although private, there was no cost to me.) All the staff were lovely and put me at ease. The difficult part was to sit in silence in a room of other ladies waiting for their ultrasound scans, with just a few friendly smiles exchanged.

I felt fine leaving the clinic after the first appointment. I needed to go back for a second appointment. I returned to the clinic a couple of days later for the second part of the medical termination of pregnancy. Again, the staff were all lovely and this time there was a very short wait for the appointment.

I was advised to rest. Back at home, after my partner and I had collected the children from the nursery, we sorted an easy tea and put a movie on. A couple of hours later I felt something similar to period pains. It felt like waves of pain. I put the children in bed and went to lay on my bed to try to relax. My partner was very supportive; he had come to the second appointment and we both knew what to expect. The pains became more painful. I went to sit on the toilet, then my waters had broken and, as I started to bleed, the pains passed. I did have the following day off work. I bled for the next day or so with mild pain.

The aftercare by the clinic was good and I felt supported. I started counselling to help me to accept my decision. I found it heart-breaking, I felt sadness and a paralysing feeling of guilt. Also, I felt I couldn't talk to my family. I went to counselling sessions every week for nearly three months.

It certainly is good to talk. Best wishes to anyone who is going or gone through this. I would recommend accessing counselling.

Reflections

As I was writing the above and reading the stories, it made me realise how alone women can feel after loss. In one way I knew this, as it is what I talk about all the time in my infant loss training, but reading the above brought it all back home for me.

No matter what the loss, individuals feel a sense of embarrassment, and in some circumstances, shame. How society and medical professionals respond to infant loss at times doesn't help these feelings.

In my accounts, I purposely explained the health aspect of my losses, as I am always struck by what women don't know about their own health. I especially had – and still have – very little knowledge of women's health, and research shows that many women know very little, through no fault of their own, just how society views and talks about women's health. How would you score yourself out of ten for your knowledge?

I feel embarrassed to say there were many health issues that I wasn't aware of. But as I have said, I want to be nothing but honest in this book.

I didn't know what an ectopic pregnancy was.

I didn't know how fertile you were straight after pregnancy

I was extremely surprised how much I bled when I miscarried.

Women's health in relation to loss needs to be spoken about so much more so individuals and couples know where to go for support.

Websites and helpful phone numbers:

Tommy's support: a national charity – https://www.tommys.org/baby-loss-support

SANDS: a national Charity – https://www.sands.org.uk/ 0808 164 3332

Ectopic Pregnancy Trust: https://ectopic.org.uk/Miscarriage Association – https://www.miscarriageassociation.org.uk/ 01924 200799

Practically perfect in every way

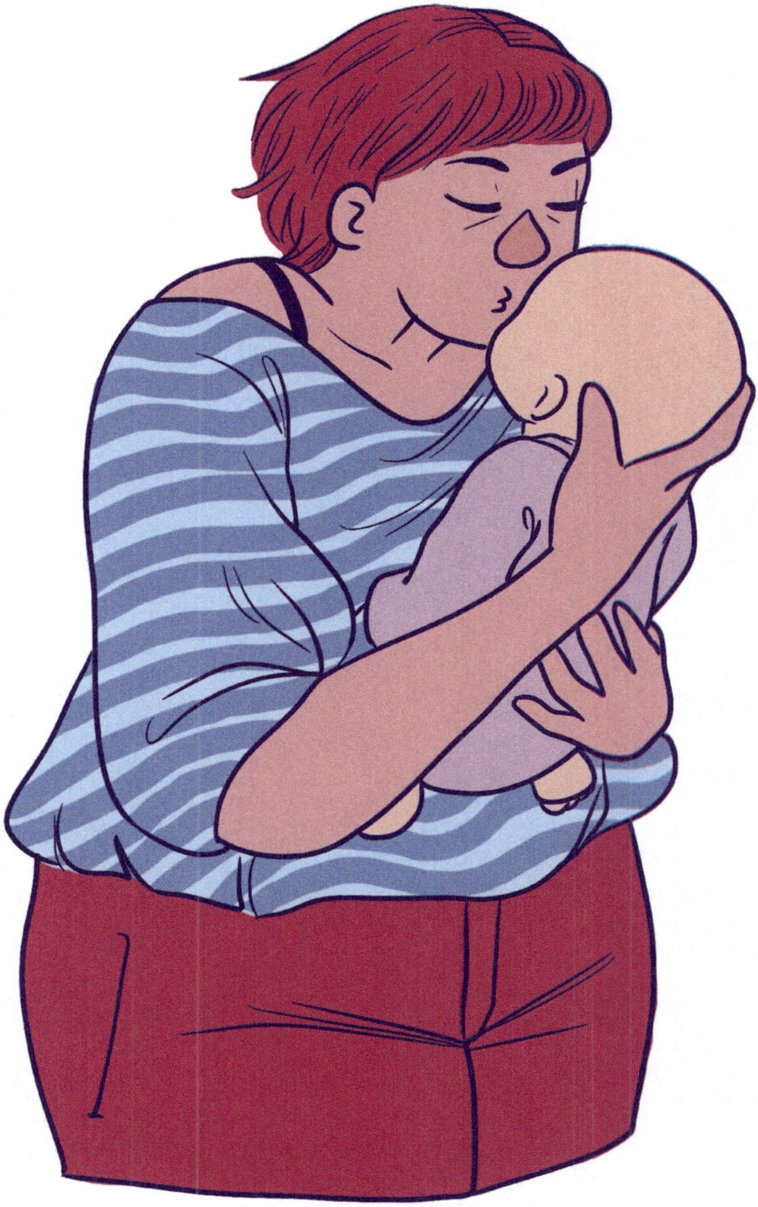

Practically Perfect in Every way - The early years of motherhood

The first two years of having a baby can be challenging in many ways – both physically and emotionally.

Becoming a mum can create changes to your relationships with friends, family, partners and other children. It can be overwhelming with all the transformations that are taking place, never mind all your hormones that are settling down.

There are so many influences that can impact how you feel in the first few years:

the support you have, how many other children you have and their ages, work commitments, the type of birth, and if there were any complications, etc.

Like my pregnancies and births, my first two years of motherhood for all three of mine have been so very different. I wanted to capture all the emotions in this book: love, laughter, pride and sadness, I definitely had it all.

Before I start to talk about my first weeks/months with my little bundles of joy, I want to include here what I have learnt is key in the first few days after giving birth.

A Sprinkle of Light to Lead the Way – Looking after yourself in the first few weeks

- *Sleep when your baby sleeps.*
- *Don't have too many visitors in the first few weeks.*
- *Be honest about how you are feeling to those you trust.*
- *Don't worry about your housework, that can wait or get others to help you.*
- *Don't feel under pressure to lose your baby weight; rest is more important at this stage.*
- *Take up help if it is offered; people like to help so make the most of it.*

Welcome to our world, Gracie Mai.

As mentioned in the previous section, I couldn't believe how beautiful Gracie Mai was when she was born – I am sure you have all said that about your own. Her dark hair, long eyebrows and how petite she was all fascinated me.

I still to this day remember the second night of being a mum – naïve I think was the word! I was still in hospital and was saying bye to Steve when I took a look at what was on television – *Pretty Woman*, my favourite film. Getting comfy, I was looking forward to watching that – not a chance! First of all, Gracie Mai needed a feed, then she had an explosion in her nappy so I asked if I could bathe her. A nurse came and supported me through it all as I was still in a lot of pain and was bleeding a lot. After her bath, I put her down and thought to myself, 'Right,

I will get to watch the film now!' No! She wanted another feed. There it was, motherhood – I was a mum.

I came home the next day and settled Gracie Mai into our family life. I am sure you can all remember that day when it happened to you? I had non-stop visitors for days and days. My dad is from a large family so all his siblings came to visit. All my friends came as well as Steve's family. Even though the midwife had said when I was leading up to my due date not to have too many visitors the first few weeks, I obviously knew better! I know many mums now are putting into place times that people can visit so it's more staggered and they are getting plenty of time for rest in between people coming to meet the baby.

After five days, I started to take my dog on walks. It was something I had done right up until two weeks before my due date. We had a massive dog who could pull on the lead so I had to be careful, but I loved taking the dog for a walk. It was my 'gather my thoughts' time. So, I was looking forward to taking him out and regaining some of my old life back.

After about two weeks of having visitors most days, I started to bleed quite heavily and was absolutely shattered as well as feeling quite emotional. The midwife asked how I was. Steve encouraged me to tell her that I was feeling quite emotional and was bleeding heavily again. Steve then told her I was also taking the dog out. As you can imagine, I was told off and told to take it more slowly. For those of you who are used to being active, I am sure you can relate to how difficult it was when told to rest.

Luckily 'visiting' to our house had calmed down. Welcoming visitors to the house (as it turns out) is quite hard work. For those of you not a parent yet, please don't feel obliged to have visitors in the first few days – they can wait!

Once Steve went back to work after two weeks, Gracie Mai and I found our own routine in the day, and once Steve was home, we had a lovely evening routine as well. I got to take the dog for a walk and Steve had some dad and daughter time. In the daytime, I took her on walks in my favourite ever pram/pushchair that took us a lifetime to choose.

Steve and I had our own business at the time so didn't have to worry too much about settling back into work. I was still able to do the accounts and promotion from home. Gracie Mai slept all the way through, and other than trying to deal with the pain while healing, I would say I adapted to motherhood well. My only fear was cot death. I was obsessed with watching her sleep, which I am sure many of you can relate to as well. I used to blow on her to get a reaction to reassure me that she was fine. I was so scared that something might have happened. When I was a teen, cot death was always in the news and I know it was developing as a fear the first weeks of being a mum. However, I was honest with my midwife and she assured me I was doing all the right preventative steps. She explained that cot death was now very rare due to the medical research that has since taken place.

Everything was good and I still say it now, Gracie Mai pretty much slotted into my life. Everyone started to tell me if your first baby is good your second one will make up for it – and no truer word was spoken! When Gracie Mai was eighteen months old, Lennon was welcomed into the world.

Love, loneliness and Lennon.

Within three weeks of being home after our very different experience with Lennon's birth, we saw a lead genetic specialist who confirmed that he had definitely got Beckwith Wiedemann Syndrome. Due to this, he was at high risk for kidney and liver cancer. I was stunned and didn't reply when the professor asked if we had understood what we were being told. I literally had no words. Have you ever been told something where no words could explain how you feel? Even so, I found words to say that I had understood and was just trying to take it all in.

Driving home, I knew we had to tell the family what was taking place but I didn't want to. Truth is I didn't want to talk about it – talking about it would make it real and I certainly didn't want it to be real. It was another mountain to climb after what felt like twenty mountains I had already climbed.

A care plan was soon put into place and Lennon was to be scanned every three months, and bloods were to be taken every six weeks until the age of seven, when the risk would significantly decrease. This was a nightmare to coordinate to start with. It took every bit of energy that I had, navigating a very complicated NHS system.

At home, I really struggled. Lennon was not an easy baby, and having two children under two years as well as running a house was a shock to the system. I felt alone and very scared. Looking back, the word 'overwhelm' definitely springs to mind. When at Alder Hey, I didn't have all this to think about; there was no housework to be done, no meals that needed to be prepared. Those that have been in the same/similar position will know that this is not by any means a privileged position to be in.

Lennon was still a very poorly baby with extreme reflux. He had worryingly started a new habit when he was crying, in that he would hold his breath until he turned blue. Every time it was terrifying and never got any easier. I felt that I couldn't ask anyone to have the children, in particular Lennon, as I didn't want to put them through the scary moments that I had to deal with. It was also easier to not go far as I always wanted to know I wasn't far from home if something did happen.

As all this was going on, I was struggling with my body recovering from the birth of my two young children. I found myself at thirty years old presenting at the GPs with pains in the vagina area and getting to the point where I wasn't confident that I wouldn't wet myself. All the glamorous points of being a mum!

The GP referred me to an incontinence clinic, explaining that because I hadn't done my pelvic floor exercises enough, my pelvic area hadn't returned to how it should! I remember looking at the physio woman, wanting to scream, "Are you kidding me?" It's the last thing that I thought about doing! So, there I was in an incontinence clinic where everyone was at least forty years older than me. Have you ever had one of those surreal moments wondering how your life has ended up here?

Every day started to become the same. I knew I wasn't happy but was somehow reassured that every day being the same was a comfort. I was in control of that part of my life, and control was very comforting after I felt very 'out of control' for most of the pregnancy with Lennon and then the first few months of his life.

None of my friends had yet had children and were out travelling, partying, etc. I felt like an outsider looking in on what my life was. I started to go to one mother and toddler group and met two good friends. I knew it was important for both the children and me to do something. We all needed to socialise and increase our social networks. I am a sociable person and wanted the children to increase their confidence with others. I felt supported with the other mothers in the group and was honest about my anxieties around Lennon. This was a big step for me. My friends explained that it was understandable after what I had been through, and more importantly, what Lennon had been through, so I felt somewhat reassured.

"It may be difficult to open up, but talking is always good. Find someone you trust and tell them how you are feeling."

As Lennon's life started to settle at home, with him now having a local GP, local physio, etc., I had a new health visitor who came to visit. She introduced herself and asked if I was OK. I said I was and smiled. She took one look at me and said, "No, you're not!" In one glance she had realised my struggles. She said to me, "It is OK, not be OK." I was so upset; I felt validated, heard and understood all in one go! It was like someone had granted me permission to be upset. I explained that I was constantly worried that Lennon wasn't well and that I didn't have the experts around to reassure me. We chatted through my anxieties and worries. The health visitor offered a non-judgemental listening ear and from that I felt so much lighter and realised that I didn't always have to hold it together. I had been through a lot – now I would go as far as saying that as a couple we had been through a trauma, which started from the day they recognised that something would be wrong with our baby.

> *It is OK, not be OK.*

When Lennon was nine months I started a part time job in a women's refuge and used to always cry on my way to work. I was due to start back at university to complete my counselling degree but soon realised that I hadn't come to terms with what had just taken place. Having spoken to course leaders about taking a year out to work on myself, it was decided that this was the best thing for me. I needed time on a one to one basis to process what had happened over the past two years. I certainly wasn't in the place to be training as a counsellor and listening to others when I had not dealt with my own feelings of shock and trauma. The fact that most of the time when I was alone I became upset was telling me I needed to do something positive about it.

I started to see a counsellor and relived the experience over and over again, until I felt I fully understood what had taken place. During this period, I really struggled at times and felt very low. I can only describe it as losing self, something I have gone on to blog about many times since. I felt my sparkle had gone, I had lost confidence and lacked ambition. To top it off, I was feeling extremely guilty that I actually wanted to be at work.

I felt my sparkle had gone, I had lost confidence and lacked ambition.

Combining these two experiences – work and studying – helped me to come to terms with what has taken place and I could slowly feel 'Kate' coming back. I was on the path to starting a new career.

In my counselling sessions, I explored my journey into motherhood and was surprised that my ectopic pregnancy also needed to be explored. What I realised was that it wasn't the responsibility of becoming a mum that I struggled with, it was more the loss of self. I am a very independent individual and before becoming a mum would basically come and go as I pleased. Before I had children, I had a job in retail as a manager, and although it was challenging and demanding, I enjoyed every minute of it. I had no other commitments and enjoyed life to the full. I'd gone from this life to feeling completely overwhelmed with commitments. I was starting to find motherhood very challenging and claustrophobic. I had been so independent with a job with lots of responsibility and great social life. From this, my life had changed dramatically. I had a job that was on much lower pay and most of the time the tasks within my role bored me. I felt patronised at times by many of my work colleagues. The only thing that was keeping me going was that I was training as a counsellor and looking forward to being qualified.

I could slowly feel 'Kate' coming back.

"Have a dream to keep you going."

Experiences change who we are. They help us grow long term, but short term it can be a battle. The counselling room provided me with a safe place to explore the past, present and move on to the future. I am aware that this may not be the support everyone needs but it helped me.

I also learnt at this stage that self-care was extremely important. You will probably by now be sick of the phrase 'self-care' but believe me, it needs to continue. In fact, when I first founded *Motherwell Cheshire*, the premise of the charity was to promote the importance of self-care and to help support mums with wellbeing activities. Self-care can come in many guises – mine is exercise.

A Sprinkle of Light to Lead the Way

- *Do an activity that you enjoy: reading, swimming, baking. It doesn't always have to be about resting!*
- *Don't underestimate the power of a good film, a bath or music.*
- *Don't think of self-care as being selfish – it certainly is not!*
- *Tune into your breath – the power of your breathing can help you get out of many situations.*
- *Fresh air always helps, no matter what the weather and no matter for how long.*

Third time lucky with Dylan James

When Dylan was born, Gracie Mai was five and Lennon four. Although he had a short stay in hospital when he was born and missed his first Christmas, I felt so different as a mum this time round. I was more confident, content with life and enjoying motherhood.

Life was quite busy as I had school and nursery runs to do most days, but I enjoyed our days together. We went to many toddler groups and activities and had a lovely routine together.

Dylan was born in the final couple months of my counselling diploma. I managed to get my assignments in and had completed my counselling hours. Other than the certificate being issued, I was now a qualified counsellor, something I had been working towards for many years.

While on maternity I got down to setting up my private practice, designing my logo, my website, etc. As I write this, I am thinking many of you will be wondering how could she do that, how selfish, enjoy your time with baby. I was enjoying time with him. It was because I had another focus alongside motherhood that made me enjoy it even more. I had learnt from having Gracie Mai and Lennon that, for me, having a focus and doing something that felt like 'me' was important to my mental health.

When Dylan was four months old, I went back to work eighteen hours a week. This was both a financial decision and a decision I knew was right for me. My work patterns were six hours – 9am till 3pm – but could be flexible around school pick up and drop offs if needed. Work was great and I appreciated having 'keeping in touch days' before I returned to work. As a result, going back to work felt a lot less daunting.

The balance of part time work and being at home with Dylan and then being at home at weekends and evenings with all three really worked for me and I am forever grateful I was given this opportunity.

Just like pregnancy, the first twenty-four months of a baby being born can impact mums in many different ways. This can be because of hormones, the birthing experience and the support that you have around you.

Here three mums explain their experiences.

Rediscovering myself – Nic's story

It's difficult being a parent. Nobody ever really prepares you for what is about to happen. When Max was born, things were brilliant. When he was eight months old, I went back to work, and Jay and I worked separate shifts, so we didn't have to pay for a nursery or a pre-school or anything like that.

When we came home from the hospital with Max, instead of us both working part time, Jay got a full time job so I could be at home with Max, which was brilliant, because I love being with him. He's my whole world. But I kinda got stuck in a rut and all I did was change nappies and do load after never ending load of washing. I became just 'Mummy'. I wasn't me anymore. I didn't have much adult conversation outside of Jay and my parents, and I didn't have any friends around because most of my closest friends didn't have children.

Max started nursery school when he was two so he could socialise and see other children, and that was when he brought home a stomach bug. That started a very rapid decline in my mental health, as well as my physical health. The fear of a stomach bug made my anxiety much worse and I was off work for over three months, although I never caught the stomach bug. It was during these three months that I decided I wanted to move home and be closer to my parents. We looked at all our options and Jay managed to get a job nearer to them so we moved.

When you have kids, you don't tend to see those people who don't have kids as much, because all your free time is spent looking after your children. When you go out somewhere, it has to be appropriate for the children. Your friends without kids don't want to go and hang out at soft play centres for two hours with what feels like hundreds of screaming kids, especially when they don't have to and they could go to Costa or Starbucks and have a nice relaxing cup of coffee. Unfortunately, as a parent, that's not always an option.

I found I was slipping into the daily grind of being a mum, and that the only reason I was here was to be a mum and to look after this tiny human. My anxiety had become really bad, to the point that I didn't want to go to those busy places. I didn't want to go to soft play or anywhere where there was a high risk of germs. I was very lucky that my Health Visitor got me in touch with a charity called Home Start (who are an amazing resource), and I had a volunteer called Hazel, who would come and visit me for about two hours each week. She would help me get out and navigate my anxiety over soft play centres and provided me with some adult conversation. For just those two hours each week, I was me again. It was about me and not just 'Mummy'. Eventually those services dropped off, and I'd developed much more confidence to be able to go to some of these places alone.

Then Max started school and I found myself thinking that I wanted to do something and make a difference, but it was difficult because I still needed to be around for Max after school. On top of this, my Crohn's disease wasn't completely under control so I worried about getting a job and childcare, and with my Crohn's, whether I'd need time off work. I mentioned in passing to a mother of a friend *from Max's class that I wanted to do something and she mentioned a charity called Motherwell Cheshire. She told me that it helps mothers with their mental health and they were looking for volunteers. I thought how brilliant it would be for me because it's the two things that I am most passionate about, supporting my local community and mental health – and that dominated the majority of my life.*

I got in touch with Motherwell Cheshire and the job was to help with Marketing and Social Media, which I could do in the office or at home. I had been helping with the school PTA and had got their Facebook page off the ground, making images to grab attention, so the position seemed perfect. The PTA work was fab, but it all stemmed back to being a mum and mum duties. This opportunity would allow me to help someone else outside my family unit. I had an interview/informal chat and it worked out brill. They were happy for me to come on board and I've been there nine months now. I feel more like me again and not just here to be a mum for Max. I have a purpose. The job I do is a volunteer role, it's not something I'm paid for, and I do it just for a few hours each week. That allows me to be that other person.

My role has led me to meet other people who've been in similar situations to me and have also suffered with mental health conditions. They have also had issues with losing their identity and have felt like they've become 'just a mother'. They've come out of the other side of it though. They've come out of the young family stage and are facing new challenges with the menopause. They want to pass on help to young mothers and families using their own experiences. It is brilliant because there is always such a diverse group of people and there is always someone who has been through what you're going through and can reassure you that you will come out of the other side.

It made me realise that the stigma related to mental health is because we don't talk about it enough. Once you start talking, others will too, and you will find more people have been through it than you can ever imagine. For example, over the summer holidays, Max and I met with one of his friends. I don't know the mum overly well, but we had time to chat, and she disclosed that she had suffered from PND (postnatal depression). It came as quite a shock to me because this person is so well put together. She is a very successful business woman and always seems to juggle work and family like this is what she was born to do. Some people are just better at hiding it than others.

> It made me realise that the stigma related to mental health is because we don't talk about it enough.

People can lose their identity of who they are, especially mothers who aren't working, and there are so many things that you can do to claim that identity back. You could volunteer somewhere for a couple of hours, whether you use skills you already have, or if you want to get out for a walk and deliver some leaflets or volunteer with an RSPCA shelter or kennels and walk the dogs or help clean them out. There are loads of charities that you can help out, like baking cakes for a bake sale. This also gives you the opportunity to go and meet new people.

Be who you are. Be more than mummy. You are a person in your own right and it's time we claim ourselves back, however that may be. Speak to friends, see what they do, see if they need help and if you can do something together.

If you can, find something you're passionate about that can make all the difference. I don't regret for a second doing my volunteer work and I've even taken on more tasks and responsibilities since I began because I love it so much.

Don't get me wrong, my mental health is still my biggest challenge every single day, but I fight it because I have to. I'm not just 'Mummy' any more. I'm me and I do things to help myself and other people. When I discover someone I've been in contact with has managed to get some help because of me, that sense of satisfaction can turn my bad day to a brilliant day.

If you're starting to feel like you've lost your identity, you can do something about it.

Spoonful of Love from Nic

"Go out there and grab the opportunity, and don't ever feel alone."

Newborn challenges – Marie's Story

I don't even know where to begin. Life has so many doors and pathways and mountains to deal with that I feel mine is always in a spiral and out of control.

I felt sadness for many years on and off when I was growing up and becoming a teenager then an adult. I don't think I realised then that I was ill.

Fast forward to being married and pregnant with my first child and realising that I was not going to get the support I thought I would get from the closest people to me. My hubby tried his best but he was new to this. If I had known I was becoming ill, then it would have made sense. From thirty weeks until forty-two weeks I did not work while I waited for my daughter to arrive but also for the mother's love and instinct to arrive too. I didn't tell anyone that I didn't feel it and that I felt empty and alone as I didn't want people to think there was something wrong with me.

I had a traumatic labour and birth and struggled to bond. There were many complications along the way for both baby and I. I woke from an emergency c-section feeling nothing for my little beautiful bundle that was my daughter. I tried to feel the bond, I tried to breastfeed. Having carpal tunnel made this difficult for me. I pumped and bottle fed but felt such a failure every minute of every day.

I went through the motions and lived the life of a mum with her first born. I did love it and I loved my daughter, Louise, but I didn't feel the glow and pull of being a mum. I found it hard work and draining. I thought maybe I needed to get back to work and then I would be OK. It was returning to work that made me realise that I was ill and needed help. I went back off work whilst I spoke with my GP and was referred for medication and also therapy. The long wait for counselling started and I chose to try the medication.

My mother-in-law had stepped up more than I ever expected of her. She had her first grandchild and was over the moon. She helped with her when she could and had her overnight once a week. She built up her skills of having a baby around again and loved the time she had with her. Even to this day, she loves having them both and adores both the kids. She is worth her weight in gold.

I learnt to ask for practical help in other areas from my parents as this was all I would get as they don't offer their time unless it suits them. I still found it hard to accept, despite telling myself to accept it. Anyway, I finally started medication and learnt to live with my mental health. I adapted my job so it was better for me but ended up finding a job closer to home so less travel and more time with my little girl, which helped me to bond more with her. I began to enjoy being a mum slowly and found ways to adapt to life as a mum and wife. It's hard to accept the new way of life with this little person who is solely reliant on us to keep them safe and well.

I found groups to go to where I could talk about my struggles and it was at one of these I met the most amazing woman who went on to open a charity to help women, girls and mothers. I volunteered for a charity but soon moved to help this lady and set up a group for mums. This helped me realise I could manage another child and also helped other mums realise they too can have their dream of more children and not let their mental health take control of their choices.

I became ill during my pregnancy with my little boy but I was ready and prepared this time. I left work and focused on my mental wellbeing and making sure I was well enough to have this child and cope with my daughter too. I used one to one midwife services and they made it all so much better and more manageable as with my first I never had a set midwife, which made it hard.

Having my midwife visit me at home so we were all involved in the checks was amazing. Louise got to hear the heartbeat and help with little things. I built up a great rapport with my midwife, Kelly, and she was amazing. When my mental health took a dip, I was visited by the midwife who was trained in mental health support and between us we found groups I could go to and therapy was set up pretty quickly due to being pregnant. This helped me get into a better place mentally and I finally felt excited about having my little boy.

It made me sad at times when I got excited as I realised I'd never felt this with my daughter. This guilt affected me for a long time as there were moments I had forgotten due to not being well. Over time, the memories resurfaced, which was nice as I could see and feel that I was a good mum for her and not the terrible mum I thought I was.

As a family, we prepared for Matt's arrival. My mother-in-law came to some scans with me and one of them was to confirm we were having a boy. She was over the moon like we were. She was going to have a grandson alongside having a granddaughter. It was lovely to see her joy and excitement. We were all excited about Matt, which was great.

I met with an amazing consultant as I wanted to aim for a home water birth and have the labour I had always wanted. The consultant and his team were brilliant and got everything prepared for me and my home birth.

I always had a feeling he would arrive earlier than expected and when I had the spotting and the twinges at thirty-seven weeks, I knew it wouldn't be long. It was 10pm on the 27th June when I felt and heard a loud pop whilst sitting on my birth ball. When I stood up I said to my hubby to go upstairs and get the flooring sheets as I thought my waters had gone. Bless him, he started to flap with joy and worry.

I called my midwife but got my buddy as Jo was on annual leave until 30th June. I was told to relax as much as I could as it can take a while to get going.

We picked the mother-in-law from home so she was here for Louise just in case. The pains came quick and fast and I felt like he was moving like Lily did to go back to back. The contractions were close together. I called the midwife back and hubby took over explaining we had no water pool ready as we were early and labour was happening fast.

Two midwives arrived and the pool was set up and I got in the water. I am good for pain and can handle it but I was struggling a lot and using gas quickly. I asked for a check and was told only my front waters had gone and I was only 3 centimetres plus he was turning. I felt something was not right and said I needed to go to the hospital. An ambulance was called, and due to not liking masks over my face, I had no pain relief, so I became quiet and coped with the pain.

Arriving at the hospital with my hubby and two midwives, I was assessed and so was Matt. He was turning and his heart rate was low. They said the placenta was not working well. They wanted to burst my other waters and I said no. I also wouldn't lie on the bed. I found my voice and went with what I needed.

I was prepped for theatre as was my husband and it took some time to get the epidural done due to my contractions coming fast. My poor midwife was sitting by my feet, listening to Matt and telling us the heart rate. Still no pain relief and my waters finally went; the poor midwife got it on her. She was great about it. We finally got the epidural in and hubby arrived.

All I remember was seeing lots of people outside the theatre doors and asking who they were, then seeing Matt being rushed out and blue. I stayed as calm as I could and told hubby to go and see what was happening. He didn't want to leave my side and wanted me to see Matt first as I didn't get that with Louise. I said just go, it's fine, he needs one of us. I was then told the placenta had stopped working and we got him out just in time. I was glad I followed my mother's instincts and went to hospital and for the c-section.

They tried to get Matt to breathe on his own but they couldn't so he had a tube in to help him breath and took him to NICU. He was a good weight for early arrival and seemed to be strong. I was determined to get the feeling back in my legs and once I was out of monitoring and on the ward in my own room due to having no baby, I was pushing myself to get to Matt. I had my shower as advised and got wheeled down (I tried to walk but I was told off for being stubborn) and met my baby. I couldn't hold him but just seeing him and touching him made my heart grow big. I didn't meet him first as it took time to recover but my hubby and daughter and brother and mother-in-law did, and knowing he had that love around him helped me.

Anyway, back to Matt being born. He gave me a more positive birth experience and despite struggling mentally still, especially with two kids, I loved it. I am who I am because of them and I would not change that. Life is hard and motherhood has not been easy for me, but I continue on the motherhood journey.

No one is alone and I hope through the power of Motherwell Cheshire that others can find that help, support, no judgement, friendship that they need.

Loveliness and loneliness – Nancy's Story

The house started being full; partner home, family visiting, piles of presents, shelves of cards and the occasional bunch of flowers in a vase. The early weeks seemed busy with texts and phone calls, visiting family and friends with a new baby, and the constant need for shopping!

An adjustment from woman to mother. The many smiles used for others, even when I wasn't feeling it. However, amongst the hard hours and days were the moments I longed for, looked forward to – these were the slightest things that reminded me of the amazing beauty of the young baby and the awesome feeling of eternal love.

As the weeks turned into months (with exception to the baby's cry), the house fell silent. I began to feel very lonely – many, many hours of loneliness – and I couldn't tell anyone about it. This isn't what I expected. Motherhood can be full of realities which are hugely different to the expectations! The expectations before or during pregnancy somewhat laid the foundations for what should be happening and what I should be feeling. I expected motherhood to be amazing, which within weeks, I soon found it wasn't.

I never expected postnatal blues in myself. I'd heard of PNBlues and PostNatal Depression (PND) but hadn't thought about it. It was never spoken about during pregnancy and then just a quick questionnaire after six weeks. This was a questionnaire done by midwives, which helped identify any postnatal issues using the Warwick and Edinburgh postnatal depression scale. A major issue for me locally is that funding issues have meant that it is one of those things that has fallen between two stools and nobody currently does it. We see so many mothers struggling who would not have had such a decline in their mental health if their situation had been picked up earlier with the questionnaire.

After a few more weeks, I was diagnosed with PND. Weeks turned into months and things felt paralysing, an enormous sense of guilt and shame for the feelings

I had. I'd never felt so lonely, but I really couldn't tell anyone.

Building some courage to seek support, I was advised to go join in some Mum + Tot groups in my local town.

I never expected to feel loneliness in a room of people as I did when I started to go to Mum + Tots. I used to think they all would be the ideal space for new mums, a group of mums to welcome other mums, a place to make new friends, time to relax and enjoy adult company. I was a very quiet and shy person, looking for someone to engage with me. A simple hi would've been nice. What I really wanted was someone to come sit and chat with me – but nothing! I used to go home more lonely and upset than before I went.

I decided to try one more group, in the hope that this one wasn't the same. I'm glad I did; it was very welcoming with many kind, friendly faces and conversations.

Motherhood can be full of self-doubt and self-reflection. I'm still not where I want to be as a mum, but the biggest thing for me was accepting that my expectations were misguided and realising the realities, as well as opening up to my immediate family about my struggles.

I've learnt a few things on this part of my motherhood journey. I'd love to share with you in the hope they will provide support.

A Sprinkle of Light to Lead the Way by Nancy

- *Loneliness is a feeling; feelings can be temporary, not depicting your entire life, simply a moment in time.*
- *Feelings can become overwhelming, therefore don't always mirror your current situation.*
- *Seeking support from others can give a new sense of self-worth.*
- *Noticing emotions when they arise can help you to observe, both how you are feeling and the situation, in order to look at how to address the issues when they arise.*
- *Remember that the current situation is not your final destination.*
- *Accept that your expectations or predictions of how things would be is not how they are.*
- *Over-thinking or worrying can add negative thoughts to a time which is already a struggle, and this could add more issues!*
- *No mum has it all figured out. There is no perfect happy family life for anyone, simply the perception some give. Trust that this isn't their reality!*

Reflections

The first twenty-four months of giving birth can be the most difficult time for many mums. Our hormones need to settle down. We need to adjust to being a mum, no matter if the baby is the first, third, fifth, etc. Every pregnancy/ baby brings their own challenges, both positive and negative. Every time a baby is born, so is a new mum. It's so important you look after yourself and offer yourself self-care. There is so much to think about, which can come with anxiety of the overwhelming responsibility that you now have.

I also wanted to go back to the questionnaire that was mentioned above. Locally, at the time of writing, this postnatal questionnaire is not being asked to be completed by many midwives. Due to changes in funding in health, no statutory organisation is taking the lead on asking for the questionnaires to be completed. As a charity, we see so many mothers struggling who would not have had such a decline in their mental health if it had been picked up earlier with the questionnaire.

Not everyone enjoys this stage, particularly the newborn stage. It's a myth that you will instantly have a bond with your baby. However, if this bond never appears as the months go on, it's important that you reach out to people who you trust.

This stage in the mothering journey can be one of the most difficult, with many emotions to deal with, and these emotions should not be dismissed as they can be something far more serious. I felt that it was important to mention the signs of both postnatal depression and post-traumatic stress disorder.

I wanted to include the following signs of postnatal depression and signs of post-traumatic stress disorder in my book as it is something I have had conversations with new mums about many, many times over the years. There are similarities between postnatal depression and post-traumatic stress disorder from birth. I hope that this helps you with distinguishing the difference. Should you feel you can relate to any of the below, it's important that you see a GP or Health Visitor/ Midwife to talk it through.

Signs of Postnatal Depression

Crying a lot of the time

Unable to sleep even when extremely tired

Expressing feelings of shame and hopelessness

Drastic mood swings

Unable to concentrate

Signs of Post-Traumatic Stress Disorder

Flashback of the traumatic situation

Intrusive thoughts or images

Nightmares

Trembling

Irritability of aggressive behaviour

Websites and helpful phone numbers:

PANDAS: A national charity supporting Post Natal Depression – https://pandasfoundation.org.uk

Make Birth Matter: A national charity supporting birth trauma – https://www.makebirthbetter.org

Resources on Government website: https://www.nhs.uk/mental-health/conditions/post-natal-depression/overview

Birth Trauma Association: A national charity – https://birthtraumaassociation.org.uk

Slips like sand through feet

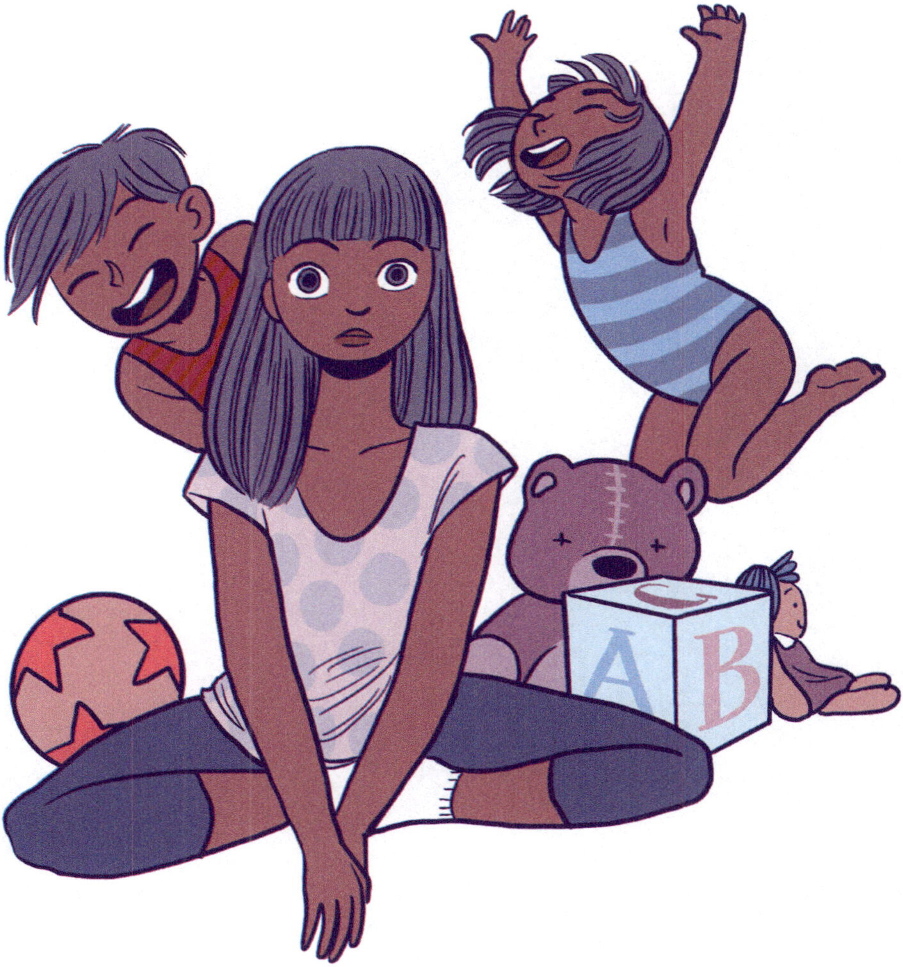

Like sand through feet – The school years

This chapter refers to what I call 'the bit in the middle' – the school years, the activity years, the working years, and for many families, the years where finances can be very tight.

As I write this book, I would say that I am still in this stage but slowly leaving. This stage is what I call 'The treadmill of life' – same shit, different day. Sorry for the swearing but that is exactly how I have felt for many months – well actually, years.

> *'The treadmill of life' – same shit, different day.*

There is so much that I could and want to include in this section. For me, it covers the many years from when Gracie Mai started school aged four till now, Gracie Mai aged sixteen years – but don't worry, I am not going to go through each year! However, I will address the topics that have impacted me over the years and the many conversations I have had with other mums in the counselling room and with mum friends. I have split this chapter into sections – easier to read and easier for me to write about!

Childcare

I have added this topic into this chapter but it could be that childcare is considered a lot sooner for many. There is simply no right time for you to consider childcare. It's when you feel ready, and for some like me, when finances dictated I had to go back to work.

Having family living near and who can help with childcare is something else I will be forever grateful for. Most of the childcare while our children have been growing up has been through grandparents, which has helped with finances, as well as finding trusted people to look after our children.

It may be that your partner stays at home and you go back to work full time. There are many options available, and like I have mentioned previously, you do what works for your family. I explore more about being a working mum in a chapter later in the book.

Nurseries/childminder fees are extremely expensive and as I write this book there are many campaigns looking to change this. I would definitely recommend doing a 'better off' calculation on reputable websites before you make the final decision of what is best for you.

Choosing childcare

Childcare is such a difficult decision to make. Every family will have their own requirements. Here are some pointers of what you many want to consider but you should always trust your gut instinct:

Questions to ask yourself about childcare

Location – *Is it somewhere that you can get to in the time that you have on your way to work? Is it accessible for others that may have to pick your children up for you?*

Hours – *Does the childcare provider offer childcare at the time that you need? If you work shifts it can be more difficult to get care to suit the times that you need.*

What's the staff turnover like? *I always think if they have long standing staff it is an indication of a setting being good. Also, having continuity where possible for young children is important.*

Meals – *What are the meal options? For many, dietary requirements are important, especially for small children.*

Security – *What security processes does the facility have?*

You will also have your own priorities that you may want to consider. If it's important to you, make sure you consider it.

"I would always say visit the care setting to get a feel for it and ask any questions that you may have, no matter how trivial you feel it may be."

Going back to work

For many, looking for childcare is usually at the stage that mums decide to go back to work to a job that they were already in or starting a new job.

In my counselling room the anxiety linked to going back to work comes up time and time again. In the past, I have run workshops on the subject. Here is what I explore in my workshops to prepare mums when starting to go back to work. I will also explore more about mums in the workplace in my 'Mums in Leadership' section.

A Sprinkle of Light to Lead the Way – Tips for returning to work

- *Use your back to work days as a way of integrating back into the workplace.*
- *Don't forget your self-care in the first couple of weeks. Things can easily start to overwhelm you.*
- *Discuss with your line manager any concerns that you have.*
- *Have a communication plan with your childcare. You may want more reassurance in the first few days/weeks.*
- *On your days off, don't worry about other household tasks; rest and spend time with family.*
- *Use your support networks to help you get through the first few weeks. There is a lot of adjustment for everyone to get used to.*

Mum guilt

When Gracie Mai and Lennon were at school, financially things were tough for us at home and I had to work many different shift patterns as a support worker in a homeless hostel to keep the money coming in. Steve worked hard and some weeks we were like passing ships in the night. Out of the school mums, there were not many of us that worked, and even fewer of us that worked long shifts like I did. Yes, mum's guilt was there, well and truly. But I did love the job; it was the anti-social hours that I didn't like.

By the time that I was pregnant with Dylan, I had moved to a 'daytime' job but was completing my counselling qualification in the evenings, so it was still difficult at times – I certainly don't do things by halves, but it all was leading to greater good!

Not wanting to sound Miss Perfect, but despite being so busy, I always made time for family. I have always done activities with the children, as mentioned previously. I felt socialising for all of us was important and I loved seeing how much they all enjoyed the activities.

Mum guilt appears throughout the mothering journey. For me, it was at this stage of going back to work that it really took its toll, and I look back now and reflect on situations so differently.

A Sprinkle of Light to Lead the Way – Dealing with Mum guilt

- *Don't compare yourself with others; we never know what is going on behind closed doors.*
- *Remember that social media is not a true story of someone's life.*
- *Tell yourself why you are doing what you are doing when starting to feel guilty – it always helps me now.*
- *Surround yourself with positive people and explain your worries to them.*
- *Write about your concerns and guilt. I always find that once I have written them down and read them out, they have a very different meaning.*

Work life balance

I have always worked many hours and always been committed to whatever job that I do. I had tried to change this but now accept this is who I am. I just have to make sure I check my hours for the week coming up and have a strict routine – sounds boring but it works for us. I also write everything down. If I don't, I honestly feel like my head is about to explode – dramatic, I know! I have notepads for every project that I am working on. God, I love a good notepad! I do this

> *When you decide to go back to work, it is another hat to wear, another role to play.*

to stop becoming overwhelmed. If I had everything on one big list, I would seriously not know where to start.

When you decide to go back to work, it is another hat to wear, another role to play. Going back to work can cause so many anxieties.

A clear routine at home is crucial for all of us as a family. We work as a team and everyone knows where they stand! I talk about this more in the next chapter – 'Mum in Leadership'.

Overwhelm

At times, despite my notepads and my self-care routine, I get stressed, but not very often. To be honest, I would say it's overwhelm that I struggle with, and it always seems to be school activities and school communication that tips me over the edge – the random texts and emails that schools send out really do get too much for me! I am sure many of you can relate? I counted the other week how many texts and emails I had received. In one week from two schools, I had eighteen emails and ten texts. All which had an action attached – and as many of you know, money expected for most as well. I find the whole thing frustrating.

As I write this, my boys do the following activities:

Dylan – football training twice a week, one match and scouts.

Lennon – football training twice a week and a match, explorers and Duke of Edinburgh preparation, etc.

Gracie Mai doesn't have any activity commitments, but either Steve or I spend a lot of time dropping off or picking her up, from her job or meeting her mates

– Taxi of Mum and Dad! I worked it out the other week that I can spend on average three hours a week sitting in my car waiting. I am lucky that I am able to take the children to school every day now and pick up three days a week, but because the older two go in earlier and come out later, Dylan and I spend a lot of time sitting together in the car. I do, however, love our little chats.

A Sprinkle of Light to Lead the Way - Managing overwhelm

This is still something that I am still learning to do but I am getting better, and these practices have certainly helped me.

- *Know that you are not the only one that is feeling overwhelmed; it today's busy world it is impacting many of us.*
- *Open up to those that you trust, who can help lift you when you are feeling out of your depth.*
- *Try not to plan too much. Lowering expectations (or creating more realistic expectations) can help you in getting your tasks done.*
- *Remember you ARE enough and whatever you accomplish each day is an achievement.*

Treadmill of life

This is a phrase I use a lot to describe this stage in my life, and a lot of mums completely agree that it sums up how we feel day to day. Same week in, week out. I long to get to Friday each week as I literally don't have a minute Monday-Thursday. I often feel a real bore as I can't be very spontaneous because our lifestyle doesn't lend itself to that. I am like a woman possessed on a Friday evening, getting everything washed, so that they can dry by Saturday to be ironed on a Sunday. Everything has to be regimented so that everything gets done on time. Even writing this. I know it sounds extremely boring! But things would just not work in the week if we were not so organised. I still seem to forget school activities, money for trips, etc. The oldest two have learnt to get the forms ready themselves and fill in what they can, then just ask Steve or myself to sign the form – and of course, somehow find the money to pay for these things!

> *I am like a woman possessed on a Friday evening, getting everything washed.*

Relationships

In this section, when talking about relationships I mean all relationships: partners, friends and family. All of which are so very hard to maintain when life is so busy. For my family, I am thankful for group chats that we set up during lockdown. Not sure how we ever communicated before! Even if I haven't been able to see family members, I have been able to stay in touch and keep them updated. I use Sunday as an opportunity to invite grandparents for tea and catch up, before I work through the ironing pile that has been staring at me all weekend (the joys).

Friendships

I am so lucky that I have some amazing friends and we all lead very busy lives. I hear from many mums who struggle to catch up with their friends. Aligning time when everyone is available can at times be mission impossible! Again, thank god for social media and message facilities. This helps me get good catch ups in between meeting up face to face. I always feel lucky that I have a wide variety of friends that I class as my 'tribe'. We are always there for each other, even though we can go months sometimes without seeing each other.

Intimate relationships with partners

This is not what I am great at, but don't worry, I am not going to go into the full details of my love life! I am the first to admit I have to work at it, and at times I need to put more effort and thought into our relationship. By the end of the evening, most nights I am shattered and so go to bed early, and then at weekends, the routine kicks in, and before I know it, it is Monday again. I have learnt the hard way in my relationship and I am forever grateful that Steve has been so patient and understanding. Over the last few years, we have invested more time to be with each other and taking time out to check in with each other. I know this has become easier as the kids have become older – but in a way, it is needed more in the early years as some weeks we rarely get to see each due to the kids activities being later in the evening and Steve is doing one trip and me the other.

Keeping the spice in your relationship is not easy. I'm certainly not saying I have this part right yet; however, I have learnt the hard way and also took advice from others. I have also worked with many couples in my counselling space and there tends to be certain patterns.

A Sprinkle of Light to Lead the Way - Parenting Partnerships

- *Communicate – sounds simple but can be the most difficult thing to do when you are passing ships in the night.*
- *Don't forget to be intimate, and I don't necessarily mean sex, but having a 'date night' can really help you both feel connected again.*
- *Try and make sure key parenting decisions are joint ones.*
- *Share the parenting load – who checks the emails, pays for dinner, makes the dinner?*

Playground politics

Whenever I think of school days (and I don't mean my school days here!), my mind heads straight away to think of the playground! Or in my case, the dreaded playground! Even now, three children and fourteen years later, I am still not a fan of the playground. I am sure many of you will have your own tales to tell.

When Gracie Mai started school, I knew very few mums as Gracie Mai went to a different nursery than most. This also meant that a lot of the mums already knew each other. As I've mentioned, when Gracie and Lennon started school I worked varied shifts and so did not always take them to school and rarely picked them up so never became part of the clique that used to form on the playground. I never joined any of the group chats so was always out of the loop on many conversations. I know group chats can be a great way for many to keep updated and make friendships, but they were simply not for me. Looking back now, it was Gracie Mai's year that I struggled with the most, because of my own insecurities and not the fault of anyone else. However, some of my closest friends now are the mums from Gracie Mai's year – a classic example of a negative turning into a positive.

With Dylan's friend's mums, I am one of the only ones who has children who are older, so they look at things very differently to me. I can remember how I felt when it was only Gracie Mai so I definitely have empathy for their concerns and worries about their child, but these concerns are not something that I have with Dylan. This is because of two reasons: Dylan is far more confident than Gracie Mai was at the same age, and the fact that both Gracie Mai and Lennon have experienced the same trip, same school play, etc. I simply don't have the same emotion. I am so very proud of him and love everything that he does, and in a way, I treasure it even more as I know each activity that he does will be my very last time of experiencing it. However, the anxiety that I had around each event with my oldest two isn't there as much now.

"Remember that this stage is not forever and for many mums it is likely that your paths will never cross again."

Finances – the bank of parents

I wasn't going to add this section but decided to in the end. As I write this book, we have just come out of Covid and are now in a cost of living crisis. My bugbear is the amount of money schools expect us to find; it has not got better in all the years my kids have been going to school.

When the two oldest were at primary schools, I have already mentioned how difficult things were financially. We are in a different situation now, certainly not comfortable, but things are not as difficult. However, I always feel for the parents that get yet another letter asking for money. Recently, when the letter came home about prom, my heart sank as I knew that there would be parents who simply go over the top (in my opinion) and there would be parents who would be struggling and stressed, wanting nothing but the best for their children.

In 2020, as a response to Covid, our charity set up our Community Share Hub, which provides school uniforms, prom dresses, winter coats, etc. The concept is based on a 'no questions asked' scheme. I'll forever be thankful that we can help those who need it the most.

Here others share their stories of work/parenting/life balance.

Life as a working mum with multiple roles – Sonya's story

I was asked to write this a while ago and am just sitting down to it at 11:15 at night, whilst feeding the baby and doing some volunteer moderating. There's a saying: "If you want something doing, ask a busy person." Yes, I'm busy…and yes, I (usually) get things done!

So, what do I do? I work part time, in three different roles for the same employer. I run my own part time business. I volunteer for two different organisations. I'm a mum to three under fives (well, the eldest just turned five, but anyway!)

How does my week look? Something like this:

Monday

7:20 a.m. Get all three boys dressed + fed. Make packed lunch.
8:30 a.m. School run.
9:15 a.m. Diddidance with the three-year-old.
11:30 a.m. Nursery run.
12:00 p.m. A bit of time for working at home/volunteering/looking after the eight-month-old.
3:00 p.m. School and nursery pick-up.
4:00 p.m. Play with the kids, reading homework, tea and bedtime around seven (for the five-year-old anyway!).
8:00 p.m. Working from home for two hours.

Tuesday

8:30 a.m. School run.
9:45 a.m. Playgroup with the younger two.
12:30 p.m. Working from home.
3:00 p.m. School run.
4:30 p.m. Running Rainbows.

6:15 p.m. Running Brownies.

8:15 p.m. Home, by which time the kids (except the baby, who comes with me) are asleep.

Wednesday

7:20 a.m. Kids up, make packed lunch.

8:30 a.m. School and nursery run.

10:00 a.m. Office day.

3:00 p.m. School and nursery run (unless there's a late meeting).

5:15 p.m. Take the five-year-old to his swimming lesson, followed by the usual bedtime.

8:00 p.m. Working from home.

Thursday

7:20 a.m. Get the kids up, fed and packed lunches made.

8:30 a.m. School run.

9:45 a.m. Rhythm Time for the youngest two.

12:15 p.m. Home and amuse the three-year-old and baby.

3:00 p.m. School run (again!).

4:00 p.m. Gymbobs.

6:00 p.m. Volunteering for three hours and maybe work.

Friday

7:20 a.m. Get the kids up, make packed lunch.

9:00 a.m. Swimming with the three-year-old.

11:30 a.m. Nursery drop-off.

12:00 p.m. Baby to swimming lesson.

1:15 p.m. Downtime or working from home.

3:00 p.m. Final school and nursery pick up for the week!

4:00 p.m. Play/food/bedtime, etc. for kids.

7:00 p.m. Work until bedtime.

Saturday

10:30 a.m. Dance for the five-year-old.

12:30 p.m. Amuse the kids until the usual evening routine.

Sunday

9:45 a.m. Church (if we can!) and be mum, then…

9 til midnight Volunteer

Start over!

To add to that, my husband works nights, so is out 9:30 p.m. – 8 a.m., or if he has an early start (usually at weekends), he's out from 6:30 p.m. My eldest is under a physio, so has exercises to do as well as the reading homework from school. My three-year-old is under a paediatrician, Speech and Language Therapy and a dietician, so lots of appointments.

I'm definitely a busy person. It may seem strange, but I'm keen to take on more work! And yes, I feel guilty. Guilty for not being at home more, guilty for not *always engaging at home, guilty I'm not there at bedtime on Tuesdays, guilty that with three, none of them get quality individual time, guilty that if one of my kids needs me I drop the volunteering, guilty that if the baby needs feeding, he still comes into work to be fed, guilty that I try to leave work in time for the school run. I've concluded feeling guilty is a big part of being a mum!*

It won't always be like this – they will all go to school soon enough and then I'll have more time to work in the day, more evenings free to be Mum. Perhaps it'll be a better balance, or perhaps there will be more to feel guilty about?

I will never regret my children; I'll never begrudge the time I spend with them, but now that I'm working, I also don't intend to give that up again. When I started working in my variety of roles, paid and voluntary, I found myself again. I wasn't just 'Mum'. Not that 'just' Mum isn't OK, but I'd done that and lost who I was, and now I've found myself again. Not a complete me – a very fragmented, multi-faceted me; I have to be as a big part of me has to stay 'Mum', but a me I can live with. A me who is busy, guilty, and getting on with life. Who worries that perhaps work means she'll miss bits of being a mum, but who knows that to be a really good mum, I have to be 'me' too!

Can you feel lonely when you're not alone? Yes, as being alone is not the same as feeling lonely.

Being a mother, I am now never alone, mainly as there's that new bundle; with this new role, many responsibilities came too, spending the days caring for another. Even though you aren't alone, loneliness can start to fill your time and your thoughts – you are not alone in this, it is normal, other mums feel it too.

Spoonful of Love from Sonya

“*Motherhood can be full of loveliness and loneliness.*”

Colouring outside the lines – Natalie's story

At school I was mostly extremely compliant. Acquiring gold stars and validation felt important.

I remember feeling very sensitive about reprimands. Shrugging them off wasn't an option, so when I was told to miss playtime in primary school for setting up a choir behind the sheds and holding my own very biased auditions, which created some bad feeling (don't ask), it left an imprint.

Amidst the need to colour within the lines, there were moments of unstoppable force (when it came in permissible guises) – like setting up a school newspaper with friends at the tender age of ten, and happily staying late to staple copies and finalise the editorial schedule.

I see now how, behind the sensitivity and safeness of 'being a good girl' there was latent boldness – sometimes fierceness – that felt incongruent but important.

Parenting has really shown me my own pervasive conditioning. My kids are largely 'well behaved' at school, though, when pockets of rebellion flash up, I am both frustrated and delighted in equal measure.

One has acerbic wit and disdain for the pedestrian. He cannot tolerate 'dullness' yet hasn't quite learnt to embrace the depths of emotional intelligence and nuance.

The other is wildly animated, full of wonderment and strident around matters of unfairness and injustice. She holds me to account against my own proclamations and reminds me daily that "Well behaved women rarely make history."

Don't get me wrong, I think there is a solid case for systems and codes of conduct. Respect and integrity are paramount. However, our learning establishments can sometimes seem rigid and immovable. I would like my children to know boundaries, but to harvest a healthy curiosity that questions why things are as they are.

Challenging the narrative is important. I want to raise children who are creative and see beyond limitation (though, my goodness, they can be exhausting to parent).

And as for me, I am learning to colour outside the lines. To be bold and courageous and safe in this uncharted territory.

Reflections

There was a lot covered in this section and I honestly believe that maybe I only touched the tip of the iceberg of what mothers have to contend with when their children are young. There are so many facets to it. The name of this chapter is 'Like sand through feet', and as I write it, it's a Sunday and Gracie Mai is entering her last week of secondary school. I am afraid I need to say the old classic, "It seems like only yesterday she was starting school," but it really does. This stage can be difficult, with multiple hats, multiple demands, trying to be everything to everyone, which can lead to stress, tiredness and anxiety. I want to encourage you to enjoy it, take time out and think of you. As the saying goes, you can't run on an empty tank – and this is true for mums as well.

A Sprinkle of Light to Lead the Way – Pointers for running a busy household

Some are my own and some have come from others amazing mums trying to spin lots of plates:

- *Write yourself a list – then prioritise. Does everything have to be done this week?*
- *Communicate to others – Who can help with the tasks? Are the children old enough to help with the tasks?*
- *Set a routine – I know it can be difficult to stick to a routine, but it can help you complete tasks. I use the weekend to pay for school trips, sign up for activities, etc. Thursdays and Fridays are school uniform wash days.*
- *If you are not enjoying this stage in your life, please reach out. Don't be ashamed. If there is one thing I have learnt since setting up our charity, it is that you are never alone. There is always someone who feels the same as you. You just need to find your safe space to share how you are feeling and get the support that you deserve.*

Websites and helpful phone numbers:

Mumsnet: A national website to support mums – www.mumsnet.com

Netmums: A national website and chat rooms – www.netmums.com

Homestart: A national charity to support new mums – www.homestart.org.uk

Working Families: A national charity to support working mums – www.workingfamilies.org.uk

Family Rights Group: A national influencing charity – www.frg.org.uk

Everything is possible — even the impossible.

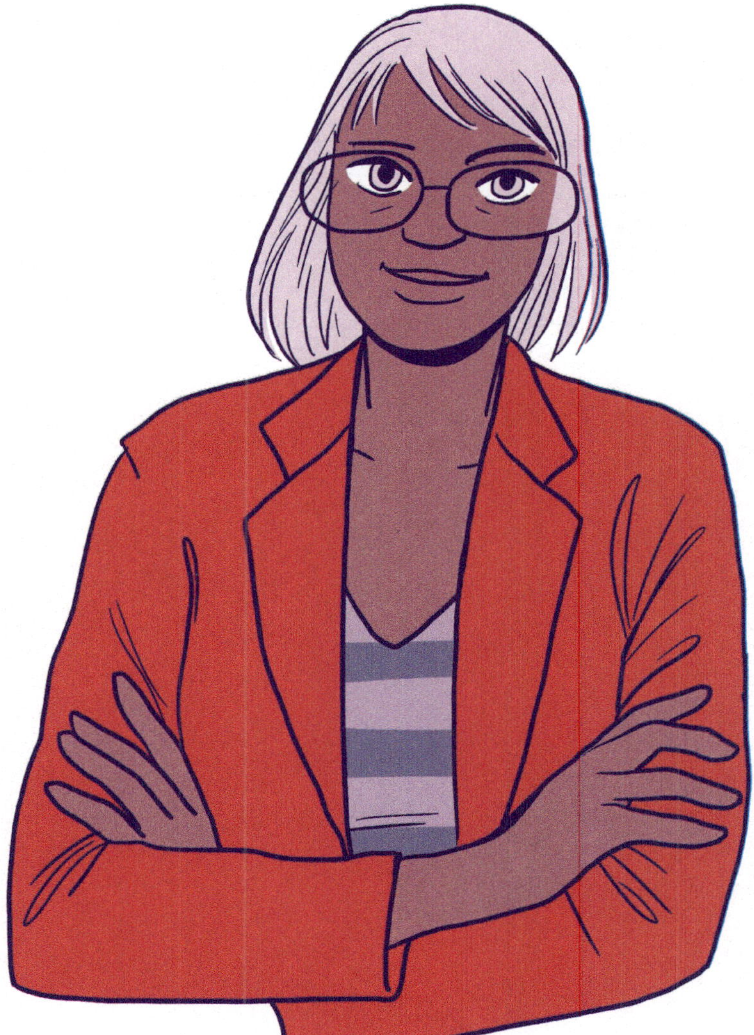

Everything is possible, even the impossible – Mums in leadership

Mums in leadership – as I write this, I am aware of how grand this sounds, and it really isn't. What I feel is possibly the best way to describe this chapter is 'mums with working responsibilities'. The mums who have responsibilities at work, which means they can't just switch off from work when they get home. The mums that can't always make school assemblies, the mums that can't always be there to pick up, the mums that would love to help the school more but simply don't have the time. We have already heard a few of the challenges linked to going back to work in the previous chapter, but now let's delve in a little deeper.

There are many of us who juggle work life and being a parent, I know, and that's why I wanted to include this section in the book.

As mentioned, when Gracie Mai and Lennon were little I worked varied shifts, but it was part time, and when at home I was at home and didn't need to think about work.

I don't know why (I ask myself this question a lot!) but I decided to set the *Motherwell Cheshire* charity up when the kids were eight, six and two-and-a-half. It was a steady start, but within two years the charity had become really busy and I was unable to keep up with the demands it required. The only way I could cope was to put in the hours or let the charity fold – and the latter was not an option. However, ironically I was not getting real wage from the charity so to make ends meet, I was still counselling. All of which was difficult. I was in a situation that I had to see through, but this caused a lot of stress at home. I felt like I was doing everything half-heartedly and nothing to the best of my ability.

Parenting: When at home I was thinking about work – Had I forgotten something? What did I need to prepare for next week? What could I be doing to help stay ahead of the game?

Working: When at work I was thinking – Had I missed anything for school? Were the kids OK being picked up by grandparents? etc.

Dylan was not in school yet. I was always thinking I should have been spending more time with him, but the time was simply not there. There was always something that needed to be done. As a friend once said, "You have created a monster." And I must admit, at the time that is how I felt. It was a case that I had got the charity this far and needed to get it to the next level. Which, by the way, meant getting funding to offer the charity more security and enabling us to recruit other members of the team to support me. This was difficult and exhausting, looking back. I put so much energy into this stage of the charity journey. It was all overwhelming, and I started to develop anxiety, in particular a driving anxiety. My head was so full that I struggled to drive to places I had not been to before. I was worried I could not concentrate enough to navigate the roads. I kept this a secret from everyone and I think for the next twelve-eighteen months I muddled through but stayed focused. Don't get me wrong, I was enjoying myself – everything to do with my *Motherwell Cheshire* journey has been enjoyable; it is my passion and I always feel privileged.

The charity has now been going for nine years and I feel that I have a mostly positive work life balance, but that responsibility has become even larger than before. I have a bigger employed team and more women and girls using our services than ever before.

I am not sure if I have become used to the responsibility that I have or now that others share the load with me, it is becoming easier. Whatever the reason, I am glad I am here!

"Find that one person that you can share your thoughts with, someone who will validate you on your mission."

To fit in everything that I do I have to be strict with myself. Someone once told me in the early years to do a little bit each day – he probably didn't mean for the next eight years! But it is very rare that I don't do something to do with work each day. However, it's even rarer that I let it come in the way of family life. Even though I love my job, what I find most difficult is that other than annual leave (and even then, at times, I have had a call) you are always at work. As a charity, we sometimes work with vulnerable individuals that can lead to safeguarding issues; as the safeguarding lead, I have to be available to my team. In the early years, I was the only one writing funding applications so very often worked till the early hours to get funding applications in before the deadline. Like for many others, the list goes on.

I know for a few years that my daughter in particular resented the charity. I think at the time she viewed it as the charity was taking me away from her – and I guess, in a way, she would be right, but it was certainly not by choice. Having said that, the charity grew fast and I was always playing catch up. I am an ambitious person and if I am going to do something, I have to do it to the best of my ability. So, after all, I guess you could say it was a choice.

A Sprinkle of Light to Lead the Way - Balancing it all

- *Find your work tribe – Who can support you on your mission?*
- *Set yourself boundaries – When do you want to work till each evening?*
- *Do you want to work during the weekend?*
- *Set priorities for the day/week – Ask yourself if it can wait till tomorrow.*

- *Make family time matter – Children really do remember this.*
- *Keep doing the things that you love – The saying 'all work and no play' is true.*

I feel very fortunate now that I have very varied hours and it works for me because I'm in control (mostly) of what I do when. This means that I can collect the children from schools twice a week and take them to school every day. I also can do a lot of the lifts that are needed.

A career and a mum – Lisa's story

A career and a mum… How do you do it? How do you have the time?

From my first day starting at primary school, I always looked at my teachers with such awe and admiration. From this point in my life, I knew I was going to be a teacher!

I would play 'teacher' with every spare moment I had: at playtime, after school and weekends. Moving into secondary school inspired me even more: the pastoral care pupils received, the extra tuition, the education in general, I loved it all. In my eyes, school has become my extended family, with teachers going that extra mile to help and support. My teachers gave me the confidence to know that I could get to where I wanted to be and achieve beyond my predicted grades. This confirmed to me that teaching was my lifelong aspiration. Meeting the careers advisor was interesting, as he said I should try out other professions. This wasn't going to happen as I was determined it was only teaching for me.

Leaving school was one of the key emotional times in my life. The five years at secondary school had been an incredible journey and one I didn't want to let go of. Moving to college was a mistake for me. I realise now that I needed the school environment and security of people who could see potential in me. Failing two of my A levels was a huge wake up call, as my path to teaching had been blocked. The same day as I received my results, I attended a meeting at the university and found a different pathway that would take me on a slightly different route but end in the same goal.

Eventually, I was on my teaching degree course, a dream come true. I couldn't have been more excited! I was finally going to get to my ambition of being in the classroom. My first placement was my best, a failing inner city school in Manchester with children with so much potential. I was able to be influential to them and be a part of their life journey. It was everything I had dreamed of, and I loved it.

Four more placements, some assignments and lectures and I was a qualified teacher. I secured my first teaching post in a challenging local secondary school. It was perfect! I had found my niche – it was working with pupils who had additional needs, either with their learning or behaviour.

After three years I moved into a consultancy role, working across the local authority, supporting schools to embed the computing curriculum. After marriage, I soon became pregnant and was so excited but was adamant on returning full time after my maternity.

I will never forget the day she was born – absolutely perfect. I started to love every minute of my maternity leave. Money became tight when Statutory Maternity Pay kicked in and I had to return three days a week when she was six months old.

It broke my heart to leave her in nursery, dropping her off crying felt like the worst time of my life, and I struggled every single day.

I wasn't enjoying my job in consultancy and was facing returning full time, so I decided I would move back to a local school. I was successful in securing an assistant headteacher position full time in a special school ten minutes away from home. When I was given the role, I cried. I didn't know how I would manage a full time pressured job and being mum. So many emotions. I was so happy to have secured a promotion, and financially this would help, but so sad having to return to work full time…but there was no other option.

> Full time work started, and separation anxiety started with my little girl.

Full time work started, and separation anxiety started with my little girl. Drop-offs were painful. I would cry on my way to work every day but my professional face was always on by the time I arrived at work, and then before I knew it, it was time to pick her up. That part of the day was magical. We then had some quality time together before bedtime and I started planning for the next day. It was hard work, I don't deny it. Some sleepless nights when she was poorly. It was a decision about who would stay off with her, both being schoolteachers where jobs would struggle to be covered – the decisions weren't easy ones.

Holidays were absolutely priceless! I got thirteen weeks off per year, but despite what people think, we still work, you just don't have the pressure of hundreds of children to look after! Both my husband and I had a quarter of the year off with our little girl. It was quality family time and was so special it made the working hours feel OK. The return after a holiday was hard but it wasn't long until we got the next one!

I wanted a second child, but I felt guilty for being a full-time working mum and didn't cope when people commented on my situation. When my daughter started school, I wasn't able to do the drop-offs or pick-ups. I had two or three mums (who were also working full time) that I relied on for information and support. When I was occasionally able to do a pick-up, other mums would often comment about me working full time: 'How do you manage?', 'How does your daughter feel about going to the after school club every night?', 'Can you not make sports day?' They weren't being horrible, they just don't think how that would make me feel…and yes, I would feel extremely upset.

Five years later I fell pregnant again. I was so excited. I had planned this one and knew what was coming, how I would cope, etc. Except the expected didn't happen. When I had my son, after about two weeks of giving birth, I quickly discovered that I had postnatal depression. My son wasn't like my first born: he didn't sleep, cried and wouldn't feed well. All my ideas and plans had suddenly disappeared, and I felt so low. I cried most days and had some very dark days. After wanting so much to do those school runs, they became hell. I didn't want to talk, I felt paranoid, sad and lonely, even though I had an amazing support network around me. I got help through my GP and started to feel better after about five months, things got easier and I was feeling more like myself. I had the return to work looming, but I told myself I had done this before and could do it again.

The second time round felt easier; going back to work helped me recover from the PND and have another purpose other than being Mum – which I absolutely loved but I equally still loved my career. I had a very supportive husband and we worked together extremely well to make sure we shared all of our responsibilities.

As my son turned four, the opportunity of a headship came up, my dream. I applied and was successful. I questioned the additional work, responsibility

> As my son turned four, the opportunity of a headship came up, my dream.

and time needed to balance all this out. It wasn't a decision that took long. I was more confident now and knew that I could be a mum and a headteacher. I would make this work!

I have been a head now for six years and never ever looked back. I have two very independent children; they both tell me they are proud that I am a headteacher and don't feel they have missed out on anything. In fact, my daughter says that she feels we have had more time with us as we have the holidays together for thirteen weeks of the year! They both help around the house, with the eldest preparing tea for the family and helping with household jobs before we arrive home from work.

There have been some low times, and there have been some incredible highs. Looking back now, I am so glad I still have my career, which is who I am when I am not 'Mum'. You CAN have a career, work full time and be an amazing Mum, you just need to be confident in the decisions you make on your pathway. I love being a Mum and I love my job!

Mum in leadership – Kate's story

I have always been ambitious in my career, wanting to develop myself and get ahead into leadership roles, but I have also had a strong desire to be a mum. I class myself as extremely fortunate to live in a society where we are able to be both – business leaders and mothers.

I have one daughter, Daisy, who was born in 2008. She was much planned after I *had suffered the loss of a previous baby to amniotic band syndrome in 2006. At the time of getting pregnant I was a communications manager at the Environment Agency, leading a small team. Whilst I was still ambitious for the future in my career, I remember thinking at the time that this role would suit my journey into motherhood more than other roles I had previously fulfilled, as it was part of a larger team and felt less pressurised. After suffering the earlier pregnancy loss, I had proactively sought a move from the private sector to the public sector for the pure fact that there was a greater degree of flexibility.*

> I have always been ambitious in my career, wanting to develop myself and get ahead into leadership roles.

However, when I was six months pregnant, the business of my husband at the time went under what became the financial crisis of 2008. My world was turned upside down and a few weeks later I found myself sitting in court declaring myself bankrupt. I felt ashamed, embarrassed, and utterly devastated. I had zero clue this was on the cards, and I was in shock.

I tell you this because it is an important context to what happened next for me in my career. I embarked on my maternity leave, knowing that I could not afford to take anything other than the minimum amount of time off with full pay. If I didn't, there would be no other income coming into the home and we would lose it. Whilst juggling nappies, breast-feeding and the general whirlwind that surrounds a newborn, I took action. That action involved a determination to get promoted into a more senior (and therefore higher paying) role at work. I put in an application and spent every spare minute of my maternity leave getting prepared. No mum

"Not having any family around me meant that Daisy was in full-time childcare pretty much from the outset."

and baby groups or watching Loose Women for me – it was leadership books and YouTube tutorials! Fast-forward three months and I was on my first day back in the office having an interview for a leadership role heading a department of sixty people. I got the job.

Not having any family around me meant that Daisy was in full-time childcare pretty much from the outset (her dad had started a new business venture). Without the support of that nursery, which was around the corner from where we lived, I couldn't have possibly succeeded in my role. Daisy will now tell me that she was always the first to be dropped off there at 7.30 a.m. and the last to be picked up at 6 p.m. She isn't wrong. But at the time I felt a huge weight of responsibility to provide Daisy with the stability of a home (something I hadn't always had as a child) and I saw investing in my career as being the only way to do that. The next five years or so were a blur of work and mum duties. Of course, every opportunity I had to be with Daisy I would be, and because my job paid well, we did keep the house and we could afford treats for her. The dreaded 'Mum Guilt' was a constant at the back of my mind, that I should be home with Daisy and not working so hard. However, I always counter-argued that narrative (which was often in my head but also sometimes vocalised by those I worked with) safe in the knowledge that my career was providing Daisy with the best start in life. She had the stability I had always craved for in my childhood. The inevitable breakdown in my marriage to her dad happened when she was five, which coincided with another opportunity for promotion at work. By then I was fortunate to have found my stride as a mum and as a leader at work. I knew I could make it work and I did.

Fast-forward to today and Daisy is a thriving teenager excelling in her academic studies, with a passion for acting that she hopes to turn into a career. Of course, it goes without saying that I am proud of her, but I am also proud of myself. I am proud that out of adversity I pushed ahead. I turned a crisis into an opportunity. Now that's what I call leadership.

Reflections

A woman can really have it all! We must not be stopped from following a career just because we are or want to be mums. The current system is clearly not fit for purpose and lots of changes need to take place for mums to have more support in the workplace. As I write this book, there are a lot of campaigns and influencing groups working to change policy and legislation. This will help more women, in particular mums in the workplace. For mums who are a leader, my advice would be to 'find your tribe'. It can be a unique and lonely place. I am lucky that my chair of trustees who I report to was a head teacher and a mum of three and so understands the struggle of trying to be everything to everybody – and how this at times is not always possible.

Websites and helpful phone numbers:

Pregnant then Screwed: Influencing charity – https://pregnantthenscrewed.com

Women's Budget Group: https://wbg.org.uk

ACAS: Advice and Mediation support – https://www.acas.org.uk

I never explain anything

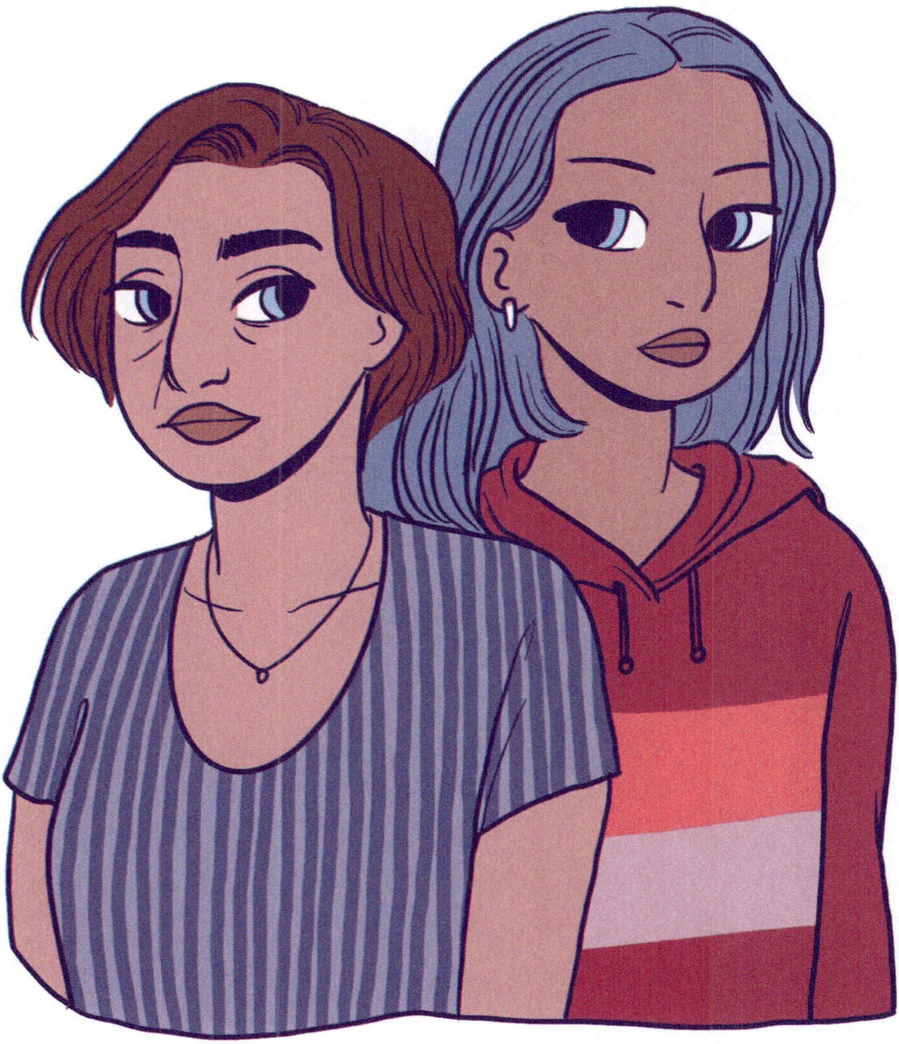

"I never explain anything" – Mum of teens

The title was chosen for this chapter as I feel it describes my two teenagers very well. Trying to get any information out of them is mission impossible!

I have reached the motherhood stage that I was most worried about – Mum of teenagers!

> *I have reached the motherhood stage that I was most worried about – Mum of teenagers!*

As I write this chapter, my boys (aged ten and thirteen years) are away for a week at scout camp and Gracie Mai (aged fifteen years) has left school four weeks ago and is never in now.

Some of the content in this chapter will link into the next chapter – empty nest.

At the moment, I am at the stage of having two teenagers in the house and a ten-year-old who clearly feels he is a teenager following in his big brother's footsteps.

This is already proving a challenging stage, but so far no arguments have taken place. As a teen, I had a lot of arguments with my parents. I was very headstrong and wanted my own independence, not always wanting the parental love that was clearly being provided. I didn't get into serious trouble at school but was never one to stay quiet if I didn't agree with something. This made for not great parents' evenings!

With all this in the back of my mind, I have been worried about the teenage years for a while now, conscious that I don't want it to become a battleground at our house!

As I write this, I certainly don't want any of you thinking I am the expert in this chapter. I want to share my own anxieties and concerns as I enter this stage in the mothering journey.

Getting the balance right

I am striving to get the balance right and just hoping I am getting it correct. In my job, the world can be a very scary place, with the stories that get shared with the charity and me. I have to take a more 'Mum' approach when speaking to the children so that their world doesn't become a dangerous place to be for them. However, I do want them to understand that they need to be street aware to keep themselves safe. For me, it's all about creating the right space for them to become independent young adults. This is done over the years and is hard work but not impossible!

Achieving the balance of protecting them as a parent versus wanting them to become resilient and learn from their own mistakes is not easy.

I would describe both Steve's and my parenting style as laid back, but I would like to think that the children know their boundaries. I am sure at some point we will get it wrong and learn from that.

“Choose your battles. Picking arguments all the time will fall on deaf ears to teens and will cause undue stress for parents.”

It is an important point for me that Steve and I are on the same page. As I say, we agree on our approach. Sometimes I can be a bit more laid back but not to the extent of anything that causes arguments between us.

I know for some parents, this can be difficult, especially if it ends up with one parent becoming the main disciplinarian in the house. This is yet another balancing act that we have to master at all stages of parenthood, but possibly more at this teenage stage. I would imagine it is incredibly difficult and tiring if you are a single mum and doing this all on your own.

In the world of social media and films, I feel our children are exposed to so much more than when I was young and so I am navigating the best way to approach some topics. I am always surprised at what they know through TikTok! But sometimes I have to remind them that what they read isn't always what is true, and this can become a battle as they see Steve and I as the old ones who know nothing. We have to remind them that we were young once – a quote that my parents used to use and I never took that on board, so I'm not sure why I think my children will.

The work-life balance is also very difficult at this stage and as I say in the 'Mums in Leadership' chapter, I am not always available when I know the kids would like me to be. Especially for lifts home at night and to and from mates' houses. And now, to pick Gracie Mai up and take her to work. Again, this is a team effort, and needs to be planned. Gracie Mai has started to stay out a lot later at parties and sleepovers. Sometimes she needs picking up when I am normally in bed, so this is challenging me on a new level – I am managing to stay up.

The magic or (lack of) on our days out.

I have always wanted my children to experience as much as possible without being spoilt, and as mentioned before, when they were little children, money was very tight, so days out were always special but on a budget! With teenagers, days out certainly are not as cheap as they used to be – a walk round a lake is not embraced in the same way as when they were small. However, I must admit it's not a 'no' to joining us just yet, but a lot of grumbles on the way.

What I do miss is the magic that days out used to bring – finding a painted pebble or collecting conkers does not excite teenagers! I loved going to the theatre or watching a film and seeing their imagination come to life when watching the storylines unfold. Whereas what I get now is faces showing no emotion as it would be far too uncool to say that they have actually enjoyed something! The excitement of something simple like watching animals in the zoo is what I loved so much about being a mum to little ones and what I miss so much in being a mum of teenagers. Whereas what I get now if I suggest something similar is "What's the point?" or "That sounds boring!" But there are still flashes of mild excitement at times.

All, however, is not lost. We are in a new phase and going for a different kind of days out now – nice meals and music concerts. Steve and I recently went to a concert with Gracie Mai and her friend. I thought she would stay with us when we got there, but as soon as we walked into the stadium, she was gone and we met her again at the end of the night. It was a different kind of night and I was very worried about her but it was great to see her at the end of the night telling us how much she had enjoyed it. I am looking forward to more days and more evenings like this. This is a new chapter for us in our days out.

In the school summer holidays we went as a family to see Noel Gallagher at Wythenshawe park. It was a great night and it certainly hit me – the kids are growing up! They all enjoyed it and were singing away. We didn't get home till 2.30 a.m. It was one of Dylan's highlights of the summer holidays.

Controlling (and nosey) mum

I am aware I can be controlling (I like to see it as organised). However, because I know what I am like, I really do try not to be a controlling mum. The battle that I have is not sorting out problems for them, but working with them to troubleshoot their problems. Actually, I am going to blow my own trumpet here; I think it's a strength of mine to develop others, and as I write this, I realise that it's actually a strength of mine as a mum as well. I think it's because I know what I can be like (a control freak!) It sometimes works in my relationship but recognising it more often than not doesn't work as a parent. The children come to me a lot for advice (which I like) and Steve and I spend time talking to them to work through the issues or troubles that they may have. They don't always agree and I have to use my inner strength to not go back at them with my opinion. We have all been there, right?

Gracie Mai now has a job and Lennon has a volunteer role as part of his Duke of Edinburgh. This has been challenging as I want to protect them. There hasn't even been issues with the roles, but I can't help but worry in case something does go wrong. I know I ask A LOT of questions when they come home each day, but I know I need to satisfy myself that everything is OK.

I am hoping this will become easier. However, realistically I know this will become more difficult before it gets better! Only time will tell.

Schools

School is another cause of stress for me, especially since mine have been at secondary school. Even though I have been more than happy with the secondary school Gracie Mai and Lennon attend, I still at times wish the school would talk to me rather than them – you know, to cut out the middle man! I do know, however, that it is important for them to develop life skills and organisational skills. What I need to develop is their communication skills as they can be very last minute and expect me to find a recipe for a spag bol at 11 p.m. Or pay for a trip that I can't afford within two hours!

I like having the old fashioned letters that I can pull out of their book bag each night and deal with it there and then! Maybe it's me that needs to change my organisational skills! Everything now is done online (my pet hate!) and so, in a way, we do get the letters, but I have to log in to read them. I guess I just have to get in line with the modern age. (Gosh, I'm starting to sound like my mum now!) Even just having five years between my youngest and oldest, I have found that schools communicate completely differently. Having portals for everything, which is my worst nightmare.

Other than parents evening – as many of you will be aware – there is very little communication with the school. This has been difficult at times, such as when Lennon had an operation on his knee and I had to email the school and explain what his mobility needs were when he started back. What I really wanted to do was to go into the school and explain everything so I had peace of mind – again, controlling. What I had to do was to rely on Lennon to communicate – which he did successfully and without me! A lesson learnt there.

A Sprinkle of Light to Lead the Way - Managing the teenage years

There are so many different dynamics to parenting teenagers, so many considerations. I certainly don't know all the answers (I'm learning every day) but these are some pointers I have picked up from others and my own experience thus far.

- *Do what works best for your family and your child. Don't feel you need to do what others are doing. Your family unit is not theirs.*
- *Phones can be a pain, but also very useful for communication and staying safe applications (Apps) Make the apps work for you family. I find them useful to know when they have arrived home from school and where they are when walking home.*
- *Compromise can be the key for a lot of decisions to be made. Involve your teen in decisions about their life; it empowers them and also helps support them when making decisions in the future.*
- *Carry out things from your side – if you say there are going to be repercussions, make sure there is. They will remember this fact for next time.*
- *Remember hormones can have a huge impact on our emotions and this can be the same for teens. They will be angry and they will be sad, but it is part of puberty.*

Teenagers are always trying to make sense of the world. Don't shoot them down if you don't agree. Listen to their opinions; it's important they feel heard.

Hormones in the home

At this time in the mothering journey there are often a lot of hormones in the house, with teens often going through puberty at the same stage as hormonal changes for mothers (and fathers!). A daughter may have started periods, which can cause lots of emotional turbulence. For boys, puberty can cause mood swings and changes in personality can take place.

Mums who may be in the perimenopause stage or menopause stage can cause their own anxieties. I would say at the time of writing this book I am very much in the perimenopausal stage, causing me to be more sensitive than usual. With teens, that can be quite demanding, and I have to check in with myself so I don't become too upset by what is being said/requested.

Over the last few years, my own anxieties have developed. At times I overthink things. My driving has been impacted (serious driving anxieties!). A lot of the time I hide these anxieties but then know it is important that the kids see that it's OK not to be OK all the time. Getting the balance right for any parent can be a real dilemma – as I see this in my practice and in the charity.

Hormones can lead to lots of difficulties in your relationships, both with teens in the household and partners: anger, being overly sensitive, emotional, high anxiety. All this can take place in one day. To make it worse, this can be a range of emotions of different people all living in the same house at the same time – no one said that it was an easy stage. Hormones certainly can cause battle grounds in the home. Luckily, it's not something I experience as I don't really get angry – sometimes though, when I do, the kids certainly stand up and listen!

However, anger can be a real issue, especially when hormones are around. Anger is not always a bad thing, but it can become an overwhelming negative emotion in the home, leading to frustration, anger, and resentment. I can find some days completely exhausting simply because of all this going on.

I remember this well from my own childhood, certainly not to the extreme but there were hormones flying around the home. I was working out who I was and desperately wanted my own independence. I moved out of the home at nineteen years old. Luckily, I had a very good job opportunity that I went to and don't regret any of it. It was the right decision for me. My relationship with my mum became stronger and on an equal level and has been even stronger ever since.

Relationships – Theirs not ours

Not quite there yet but there are definitely boys in Gracie Mai's life at the moment. On a friendship level, she claims! Since she has left school she has been going out a lot more and there is alcohol involved at some house parties. So, it was decided that we would have another 'mum and daughter' talk about the birds and the bees. I didn't really know what to say, to be honest. Gracie Mai was mortified that I was actually having the conversation with her. Basically, I just wanted her to know it is important that she is never forced to do anything that she doesn't want to, that she stays safe at all times, and doesn't drink so much that she can't remember her actions. Think I covered it all!

I know each parent has their own opinions on relationships and it is certainly not for me to offer advice and guidance. I am learning and I am sure there will be challenges, arguments and mistakes along the way.

Friendships

At this stage I find there are two dynamics to friendships at play in the family: their friends, and them becoming our friends.

I have always been lucky that my children have such lovely friends with parents that I communicate with on a regular basis. However, I know many parents who are struggling with their children’s choice of friends and this can be very difficult to manage. It can become a battleground, with both sides having opposing opinions. Young people don’t always see what we see in relationships, and as difficult as it may be sometimes, this stage needs to play out, but I completely understand that this may not be possible if there is a high risk of something risky/dangerous taking place.

I don’t want this book to become a parenting book so I won’t explore this topic much more, but have added links at the end of this chapter that may help.

However, this stage doesn’t always have to be doom and gloom; there is a good chance that your teen will become a friend. Having said that, it is important that you maintain boundaries. You will always be your child’s role model. I know from counselling that many individuals have struggled when the boundaries become blurred.

Gracie Mai comes out with me socially quite frequently; we swim once a week and go shopping together. I have not ventured on a night out with her just yet and don't really think she would want to do this at this stage!

Lennon is currently completing his Duke of Edinburgh Award and so we have been on some walks together.

It's been really lovely to spend some one on one time with them; it becomes very rare.

Whereas Dylan and I spend hours in the car together chatting and hearing the gossip of school life.

Relationships – ours

Parenting a teen can be challenging, especially when your partner has different opinions. Or for single parents, I am sure it can be very lonely when trying to navigate what the right decision should be on a range of decisions that need to be made.

As previously mentioned, I have always felt lucky that Steve and I have similar opinions on parenting, but we are now certainly entering new territory. So far we have not had any arguments or differing opinions; actually, quite the opposite, and we have pulled on each other's strengths.

In my counselling practice, I have worked with many women and some couples who have struggled at this stage in their parenting journey as their partner's opinions greatly differed to their own.

"If you're disagreeing with your partner, don't take this out on the child. Communicate with each other to find a compromise that you both agree on. Don't use the child as a pawn in the middle."

Mental health in teens

I didn't want to end this chapter without addressing the struggles that some parents may be experiencing due to their teen having their own mental health issues.

As a charity, we have the Inspire Project that supports the mental health of teen girls. Over the last three years the demand for our services has increased year on year and we are seeing young women struggling with:

Body Image

High Anxiety

Social Anxiety

Eating Disorders

What is clear is that parents are fighting to get the right support and I see parents really struggling and blaming themselves, at a loss for the right support for their child and themselves. In my experience, parents struggle to get anywhere when they are asking for help. Many of them feel like they are in a hamster wheel, going round and round in circles in an impossible-to-understand system. I can't imagine the frustration that any parent has who is experiencing such an onerous time.

Frequently, I get asked for advice and guidance from other mums who are worrying about their teen's mental health, and even though I don't want this book to become a practical advice book – God knows there are enough of them! – I wanted to take this opportunity to mention the issues that may arise, hoping it will help others who are concerned about their teen.

If you are noticing any of the following with your teen, you may want to have a conversation with them to raise your concerns.

- *A change in what they wear, e.g. always long sleeves, winter clothes in summer.*
- *A change in eating habits, saying they are not hungry, saying they have eaten earlier in the day.*
- *Not going out with friends like they used to or having a new friendship group that corresponds with a change in behaviour.*
- *The way that they talk about themselves is becoming very negative: "No one likes me anyway" "Who cares what I think?"*
- *Stopping seeing friends when in a relationship.*

All the above may be nothing to worry about but I know from other parents that they can also be warning signs. A positive and supportive conversation early on can really make a difference.

I have included charities and statutory support that are available in the contact section, but truth is there is limited support. I wish I could change it but I can't – YET! However, I do mention the struggles at every meeting that I attend to make sure family support is available.

This stage is very difficult for all involved: parents still trying to be the protectors and teens wanting to explore the world but seeing no danger. It is, however, still possible to try to understand each other on a different level. Mistakes will be made on both sides and relationships can fall apart, but it doesn't mean this stage will be forever.

The key can be understanding what they need, and what you need. It can be a really positive experience and friendships can be developed as your children get older.

These stories are from mums who themselves have their own unique stories of parenting a teen, the ups and the downs, the positives and the sacrifices.

Mum of a teen – Sheila's story

When my hair is dripping wet and I reach for the hair dryer only to see the empty socket, I remember I have a teenager across the hallway. Make up, hairspray and deodorant have become items I merely 'borrow back'. How did I get here so fast?

I had imagined motherhood, but never in a million years did I imagine my years as a mum to a teenage daughter would be as they are. I had prepared myself for the "Can I stay out late?", the sneaking out for the odd alcopop or cider, the obsession with boys, the parties and the homework battle! No one who knew me as a teenager would be more surprised than me to get my daughter to sixteen years of age without any of the above.

I have somehow found myself with a friend – a friend who needs a little guidance now and then, a taxi often and a service wash that would give the local launderette a run for their money, but no stress... yet. I say yet because life as her mum has been a pleasure (NO smug mum here by the way – I have more than one child, and the other more than makes up for it and brings me many challenges).

Calm, grounded and sensible; I find myself checking out my own behaviour in comparison. I take a step back at times and wonder how she became more grown up than me. She has, in her teenage years, coaxed the calmer person out of me too – the calming influence of my husband, her step dad, may have helped us perhaps.

I have a partner in crime to deal with the three somewhat louder teenage brothers – she delivers a harsh line, and I'm reminded she is her mother's daughter. I look and see in her a generation so accepting of others, a generation challenging small minds and banishing many stereotypes. Wow! What progress they are making!

The recent introduction of a boyfriend hasn't rocked our world; in fact, if I could have chosen one for her, it'd have been the very one she's brought home.

I should be grateful – and I am – but it doesn't stop the worry. What's next? University? I love the fact she kept her circle small and didn't seem to suffer the 'FOMO' when party invitations weren't for her, but is that grounding there for good? The night life of a university city, the walk home in the dark, the driving... Arrghh – no, the worry never ends. But I wouldn't change a thing.

Our invisible disability – Leanne's story

My daughter is fifteen and has an invisible disability. Her daily challenges and struggles require constant parenting. Due to her hidden disability, she is socially isolated and finds it difficult to go out alone.

My parenting has adapted due to her challenges and struggles and is probably quite different to 'traditional parenting'. This interestingly can bring judgements from family, friends and other parents. Judgements that take the form 'if she was my daughter she wouldn't get away with that' and 'let me have her for a week and see how she is then'. I am at a stage now where I am used to ignoring the flippant comments.

Parenting my teenager has come with sacrifices, such as giving up my career to be a parent carer as her needs became more pronounced. Simple things such as asking her to 'pop to the shop' are impossible. Every decision is taken with her disability being at the forefront.

My daughter's neurodiversity means that we have a unique relationship. A wonderfully close relationship. She has the most amazing sense of humour and we belly laugh together. I love that she is so strong minded and not a people pleaser. Her passion for fashion and eye for design never fails to amaze me.

When I was her age, I was pushing the boundaries with my parents, constantly out with friends, enjoying more independence, and had a Saturday job. I thought my challenges with my daughter would be similar, but hers are vastly different and independence, at the moment, feels a long way off. Watching my son as he approaches thirteen is a vastly different experience and I am enjoying watching him mature in his own way. I am developing skills that I didn't know I had while parenting a son on my own.

Tweens to teens: From neediness to disdain – Emma's story

You might think that this motherhood thing becomes a part of your identity, but I'm still shocked when I hear myself say out loud that I'm the mother of thirteen- and fifteen-year-old girls! I still don't really understand how that happened.

People say that it passes you by in the blink of an eye. When I was the mother of two toddlers, I wanted to thump those people! In that haze of sleepless nights, and feeling so totally lost to others' needs, I never believed that these years would end. But they did, without warning. And as much as I wanted them to (I wasn't cut out to be the mother of young children), I wasn't prepared for the transition from neediness to disdain...

My eldest had been at high school for less than a month when she told me that she didn't want me to drive her to her birthday party. The party that I'd suggested, booked, baked a cake for and organised. I tried to let it go, I tried to be adult about it, but I was so hurt, I failed.

"But why? What's wrong with me?" I wailed.

"You'll talk to them. You'll sing. You'll ask them questions. Dad won't," she said, rolling her eyes.

"I'm friendly, what's wrong with that?" I asked.

"You're just embarrassing, Mum. I don't want you to talk to them!"

Now, I am a cool mum, so this came as a complete shock to me! Maybe I wasn't as cool as I thought?

As time went on my little girl started to change. She wanted to fit in; making friends was more important than spending time with her mum. We argued, we struggled to understand each other. The bond we had seemed to be lost and I was grieving it, I was grieving her.

Then one night, I noticed how underneath the disdain, she seemed sad. I asked her if she was okay and she cried. For the first time in a long time I listened to her. My god, being a teenager is tough, and she was struggling with the transition far more than I was. She spoke about how she was confused, about how much she wanted to fit in, and how this sometimes meant that she did things that she didn't understand, that didn't seem to fit with her identity. She was going through a transition from child to young person, she was trying to find her way, and she was feeling lost. I was part of the problem; I was trying to make her be somebody she had grown past. I was so lost in my own grief that I had abandoned her.

This was the moment things changed for us. I told her I was sorry; we both cried. I explained how much I was struggling with the transition too, and that I hadn't noticed how difficult it all was for her. I told her that I was there for her and I wanted her to grow and find out about the young woman she wanted to be. I said that I would give her the space and support she needed to do this.

It's not always been easy; I've not always been perfect, nor has she. There have been times where I've felt like I don't know her anymore. But I made the decision to approach the ever-changing new parts of her with curiosity, and that's made me feel excited. Each day she comes home from school with new opinions, new passions and new friends. She's experiencing the world, and I get to have a front row seat and watch her take on these adventures with a deep love and pride, and my heart in my mouth!

She's quite a force. And I think that the teenage years are fast becoming my new favourite.

Reflections

Parenting a teen certainly can be a difficult time. There are so many considerations, especially as they go between being a child to an adult. The balance of giving them freedom and protecting them at this stage can be a difficult one.

The most important role at this stage is to be open and honest so that your children can trust you and be open and honest back. The dynamics of your relationship may change, but it is important to remember that you will always be mum! There may be some challenges ahead where you could do with a good listener to help support you.

Websites and helpful phone numbers:

NHS link containing resources: https://www.nhs.uk/mental-health/children-and-young-adults/advice-for-parents/cope-with-your-teenager

Family Live Family advice website: https://www.familylives.org.uk/advice/teenagers

Young Minds: A national charity – https://www.youngminds.org.uk/parent

Mind: A national charity containing resources – https://www.mind.org.uk/for-young-people/information-for-parents

Kooth: A national charity for young people (login is required) – https://www.kooth.com

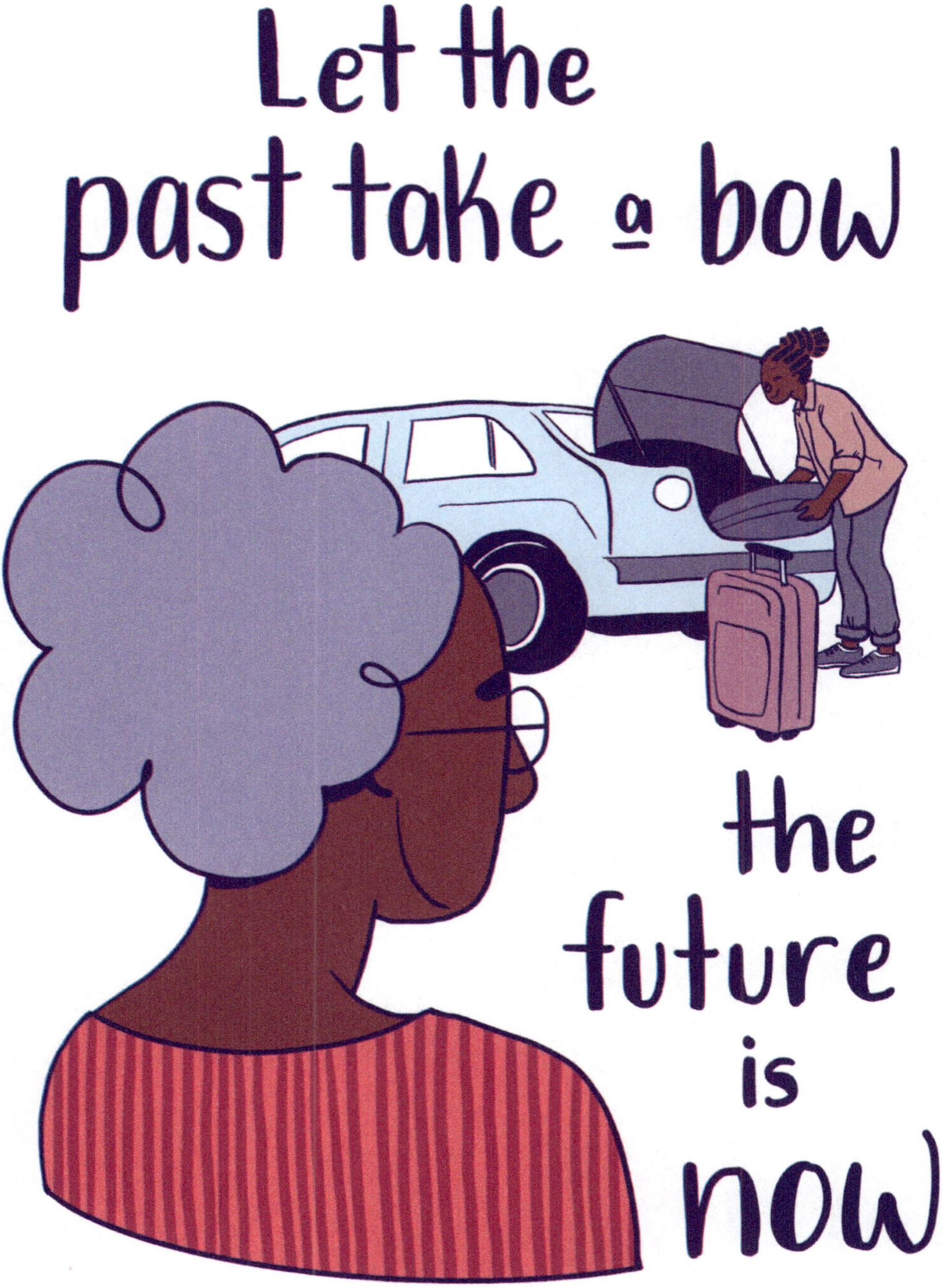
Let the
past take a bow
the
future
is
now

Past take a bow, the future is now – Empty nest

I haven't experienced the period covered in the next two chapters yet, but didn't want to get this far in the book without addressing these stages of the mothering journey. These are definitely two stages that I think about a lot at my time of life, and they are stages that have been discussed frequently in my counselling room over the years. As a charity, we have evolved to support more women over forty-five than ever before, with women aged sixty to seventy-five becoming our fastest growing age group.

Empty nest – this is a topic that is getting spoken about so much more and even GPs are talking about 'empty nest syndrome', in particular in relation to mums. Although none of my children have yet left home, as mentioned in the previous chapter, there are elements of parenthood I am missing already.

I am pretty sure that empty nest has always been there for parents, but like a lot of issues, we are now talking about them more and they are being recognised and given a name. It's a term being used for mums who are feeling lonely, very down and missing their child/children. More people are now moving away from their hometowns and this can mean for many parents that they are not seeing their children on a regular basis.

This stage in the mothering journey can be a very tough time for some and a new lease of life for others. I have witnessed this in equal measures. I plan to capture the highs and lows of this stage so no woman feels alone with their experiences.

Purpose or lack of purpose

When your children leave, a time for adjustment is needed. Particularly if you have not already prepared yourself. The loss will feel perhaps sudden and like a bereavement. You will need to identify new roles and interests that can now bring meaning to fulfil your life. You cannot just get used to these adjustments, you need something else to fill the void, especially if you have been a stay-at-home mum. Even for mums that have been working, there can be an element of questioning what their purpose is now. With the additional time that mums have, they can start to feel lonely and miss the children more than they ever could have imagined.

For others, this stage gives them the space and time they have been longing for in a very long time. I know myself I have a plan of what I want to do when I have more time – join a rambling group, start bird watching and go to many more theatre shows! Real rock and roll!

Since founding our charity and linking in with other women's groups, I have been struck by how many groups there are now, and with the power of the internet, there really is a group for everyone, connecting like-minded women. It can be a big step joining a new group, but remember everyone in the group walked through the doors for the first time once and everyone will be welcoming and happy that someone is joining their group. There are many platforms that will support you in finding groups that suit you. Social media is a great start; there are lots of Facebook groups – some really great, some not. Take a look at the group rules and the comments that are on the group to get a feel for it. Your local library is another great resource. Libraries run many groups and also promote other local groups. There are also lots of new friendship platforms, such as MeetUp and Bumble. I have heard really positive things about both.

A Sprinkle of Light to Lead the Way – Joining a group

I know from running many groups within our charity that there is a lot of anxiety when joining a group, especially when attending for the first time. Here are some tips to help alleviate the anxiety that may creep in when considering joining a group:

- *Find out the practicalities: Where do you park? What is the lighting like if the group meets at night? Do you need to take anything with you? How do you pay?*
- *Consider contacting the group beforehand. There may be someone from the group that could meet you at the door.*
- *If there isn't anyone you can contact beforehand, perhaps go a bit earlier for the first few sessions so that you don't have to walk into a full room.*
- *Check with your networks to see if anyone else is going to the group or fancies joining; you may well be surprised!*

"Loneliness can have such an impact on an individual's mental health. It's important that you keep communicating, challenging yourself and connect with like-minded people."

Relationships

For many, this empty nest stage can be very challenging for their relationship. Without the children being around and having to take them there and back to places, many individuals find that they no longer have anything in common with their other half anymore. With the kids no longer being around, it's like a spotlight being shone on this fact!

For many mums, their identity has been being a mum, and when the children are no longer around, this can be a daunting time and can have an impact on self-esteem and confidence. This, in turn, can have an impact on relationships. The spark is no longer there, the connection has gone and for many, communication stopped a long time ago but nobody actually noticed.

This, however, can be the complete opposite for others. With the children not around and far less commitments at home, this time can be an exciting new chapter, like meeting for the first time! Weekends away, walks, meals, the list can be endless.

A Sprinkle of Light to Lead the Way - Maintaining a healthy sex life

This section could be added to any chapter, but for me it seemed to fit in this stage of my mothering journey.

- *Get naked – Having skin to skin can help with oxytocin; this can help you feel more sexual.*
- *Masturbate – Either on your own or with your partner. Take your time and find how to enjoy your body in a sexual way.*

- *Spend time together – At this stage in your relationship you may be leaving little time for you to be together. Find the time to reconnect; it can simply be lying on the sofa or chatting in bed.*
- *Laugh – As the saying goes, laughter really is the best medicine. It's good for the soul and can be a great way for you and your partner to feel connected and remember what it is like to have a giggle together.*

"Keep communicating. Tell each other how you are feeling about the kids not being around. Explain what you would like to do with your extra time. Find activities that you can both do together."

Menopause

For a high percentage of women, as an empty nest becomes a reality, another life transition will be taking place. Like in pregnancy, the menopause can have a huge impact on our hormones and can, for many, go on for years. Menopause is the time that marks the end of your menstrual cycles, and just the thought of that really upsets me. It is now no longer my decision if I want to have another baby, the choice has been taken away from me. For many, this, alongside empty nest, can be another type of grief. For others, however, this can mean freedom: freedom in the bedroom, freedom from having a period each month.

The menopause is not just about our menstrual cycle stopping, there are many symptoms that can take place for women who are going through this stage in life. Menopause is a big issue currently for women, and is a big part of my work presently, with many women struggling with symptoms of perimenopause and menopause and not understanding where to go for support, and struggling with getting professionals to offer appropriate support and guidance.

Here are some, but not all, symptoms of the menopause:

hot flushes

night sweats

vaginal dryness and discomfort during sex

difficulty sleeping

low mood or anxiety

reduced sex drive (libido)

problems with memory and concentration

hair loss

itchy skin

The menopause can impact our hormones, just like when a mum gives birth, with our hormones changing literally hour to hour. Going through the menopause as well as significant life changes such as children leaving home can be an upsetting and challenging time. It's important to talk to others, and in certain situations talk to health care professionals. This is particularly important in relation to conversations regarding menopause treatment.

A new type of caring

At this stage in life our own parents will be getting older themselves and mums may stop caring for their children on a daily basis but start caring for elderly relatives. This can be a demanding and thankless role but a role that we feel that we have to do.

I have met with many individuals in the counselling room who have been carers, and my mum was also my nan's carer. It's a difficult role which can be draining and many individuals feel guilty about not wanting to do it. It can cause strains on partner relationships and also strain the relationship with the parents.

The sad reality at this stage is that for many individuals, they may be experiencing loss of their own parents Again, this can be another isolating experience. I have included some links to grief support services at the end of this chapter. I explore more about caring commitments in my next chapter.

Many women that I speak to feel lonely with no one to talk to who fully understands them, no one that they feel connected to anymore, no one that they feel they can reach out to.

The stories below all share their own stories of their experiences of empty nest.

Empty nest and me – Debb's story

I remember so vividly the warm feeling of being so wanted, needed... not having a minute to myself, desperate to have an odd day/hour/minute to myself... but knowing that you were the person your family came to for every crisis, no matter how big or small! It gave me great purpose in life. I've always worked, but nothing gave me the great sense of fulfilment that being a mum did.

Fast forward ten-ish years and how different my life is. Those days/hours/minutes I craved for are now my nightmare. How I often hate weekends. They stretch ahead with no purpose. No one to share a giggle, a pointless conversation. I sometimes think the shop assistants I engage in conversation with must think I'm some sad, lonely old woman. I crave human interaction and that's why I chat to them. On weekdays, I try to fill to capacity so I don't have to come home to an empty house – and often result in me being exhausted! But I don't mind, better than facing my loneliness. Work gives me back my purpose. Don't know what I'd do without it. I have friends who are looking forward to retirement... NOT ME!

My children are adults and have their own lives. I am so proud of them. They have grown into beautiful, independent people. They do occasionally need me. Maybe grandchildren will bring back some purpose?

Looking back, I don't think I enjoyed my time as a young mum as much as I should. Oh, what I'd give for those times. Yes, it's hard work, tiring and very frustrating but I wouldn't have missed it for the world!

I am now embarking on a new life that is full of adventures with friends and family. I have my own caravan and love my weekends away connecting with friends some weekends and connecting with myself other weekends. This time away gives me something to look forward to in the week.

Off to university she goes! – Cheryl's story

When Emily told us she was going to university I was thrilled. As it neared her looking around and deciding where to go, I began to feel both nervous and very sad. I was worried as Emily has had problems in the past and we are very close. She is quite dependent and is very often around. I was worried as she would be leaving home to live in a city she doesn't know and I wouldn't know what she was doing or who she was with. I was sad because my first born was leaving home, and although it's not far, I wouldn't see her every day.

In the run up to looking at universities I would very often get upset whilst talking to others about it. We went to look around some universities and this helped to ease my mind. We saw the kind of accommodation she would be living in and were told there is security on campus and people on hand if there were any problems or worries. Emily decided that she wanted to go to Chester. We were happy with this as it's not that far away and it's not a huge city.

After Emily applied, she had to decide what accommodation she wanted, I found this process really tough as it hit home that it was really happening. Emily got her A level results and proudly got into her first choice – Chester. By the end of that week she found out that she was going to be living in a self-catered, shared kitchen and bathroom house. This was welcome news as she would be sharing it with five other girls. The university set up a group chat for all the students on the road so they could chat and get to know each other before moving in.

The week leading up to Emily moving in was hard; I offered to help her pack but there wasn't anything I could do which upset me. She went out for lunch with her grandparents and that evening she was really quiet. It was hitting her that she was leaving. The following two days she worked so was able to keep busy. I worked one day so didn't have time to think about it, but when I did, I got upset. Luckily, my work colleagues are very supportive, which helped.

The day Emily moved out was hard. I surprised myself, though. We loaded the car, drove her there, helped her to unpack. It was only as we were leaving that I cried – lots! I cried part of the way home then pulled myself together, then got on with my day.

The first week of Emily leaving was very strange. It was odd knowing that she wasn't going to be home, knowing I couldn't tell her mundane things, such as I was with one of her old college friends that day. It was weird at night seeing her curtains open and not looking in on her before I went to bed.

We went to take her out for lunch. It was lovely to see her and we could see she was very happy; she was already more confident. She has grown into a beautiful young lady who is following her dream. Even though I am sad not to have her around, I could not be any prouder of her.

Empty Nest Syndrome – it's real! – Caroline's story

Is it possible to feel empty nest syndrome before all your children have fully left home? I reflected on this thought over the years. I told myself that it wasn't 'normal' then questioned 'Well, who made the rules?'

My husband and I have three children: Harry, James and Grace. There are five-and-a-half years between the oldest and youngest and two years, four months between the boys. Life was chaotic, exciting, fun, hard work and expensive – full of highs and lows. I threw myself into being a mum with enthusiasm and lost myself a little along the way. But I valued working part time. I changed careers and completed a degree in 2013, not long before we began university visits with Harry. Being Mum sometimes brought out the best in me and sometimes the worst in me.

Harry left home to start university two weeks after our third family house move. The first week, I felt as if I had been hit by a bus. Wham! Nothing had prepared me to feel this grief-like reaction to our first child leaving home. I asked myself, 'Why do I feel so heartbroken when I still have two children at home?' Undoubtedly, I was experiencing a rollercoaster of emotions which were heightened due to the house move. I didn't realise at the time that I was also perimenopausal. I had put enormous pressure on myself to decorate and organise Harry's bedroom, to give him a space to return to, before he left for uni; it felt important that he establish a connection to our new home before he left. Later he told me that he couldn't recall our address on uni admissions day.

When James went to uni, I didn't experience the same feelings of heartbreak. Being better prepared and with my emotions more stable probably contributed.

However, when he left home for good, six years later, it left me with feelings of emptiness. Sadness was my overriding emotion this time. I had enjoyed James' company in the three post-uni years, which also included Covid. We had got to know his girlfriend, who spent alternative weekends at our house, so it was almost two young adults leaving this time. Realisation began to dawn that we only had one young adult left and by now Grace was living at uni, eighty miles away, during term time.

Grace was in her third year of a four-year course when James left home. A few months later she broke up with her long-term boyfriend who lived in our village. Again, the strength of my reaction surprised me. I convinced myself that in finishing with her boyfriend she was also severing ties with us, that I wouldn't see her anymore; my mind was entirely occupied and overrun with these thoughts which were tearing me apart. I was grieving for her leaving home before it had even happened!

I always encouraged our children to seek independence, to be strong, find their way and follow their passions, so why did I have these strong reactions when they left home? I reflected on my emotions and eventually came to the acceptance that the bond created between a mother and her children, a fundamental part of our biology, means it is natural to feel the pain of emotional turmoil when they leave us.

Time healed my pain and I began to enjoy new ways of being Mum. Years of mindfulness practice helped me. I rode the wave of my emotions rather than suppress them; I reflected on 'Who am I?' and wrote a list of thirty-two ways I can identify myself. My children will always be part of me and now I am embracing the opportunities ahead of me. We all experience life's transitions in our own way, there are no rules or conventions.

Reflections

It is clear that this phase comes with many emotional and physical challenges that are not too dissimilar from becoming a new mum. Yet we speak and respond to the topics very differently. We nurture new mums, yet many people laugh when the word menopause is mentioned.

Something that I am voicing a lot is that there is a clear support pathway for new mums, yet women going through the menopause in many cases have to fight for the right to get the right support and medication. I am seeing health inequalities growing recently with many women who can afford to choose private health care and get the right medication, leaving those women that can't afford it struggling.

This stage can be isolating and you may feel very alone. At this stage in life, many people may feel there is no one going through the same, making it even more difficult to speak about.

However, what is clear is that there are many going through the same and it could be crucial to reach out to like-minded women. The good news is that things are changing and changing for the good. As I write this book, our charity hosts many menopause cafes. Throughout the country there are many menopause cafes being hosted, connecting like-minded women. In spaces like these, women are able to talk not just about loneliness, but also about how menopause symptoms may be impacting them, and get appropriate advice and guidance from others who have 'been there'.

We must also not forget that on the flip side, this stage in life (as I am just finding out) can be exciting and a new women can emerge, with a new tribe of friends who are understanding and have shared interests. It can also provide time to go out with our other halves more and connect on a new level.

Websites and helpful phone numbers:

Menopause Cafe listings: https://www.menopausecafe.net

Age UK: https://www.ageuk.org.uk

Relate: A relationship charity– https://www.relate.org.uk

University support: https://www.universitiesuk.ac.uk/topics/students/student-support

Meet up: lists meeting opportunities – https://www.meetup.com

Give us treats,
sing songs,
give sweets!

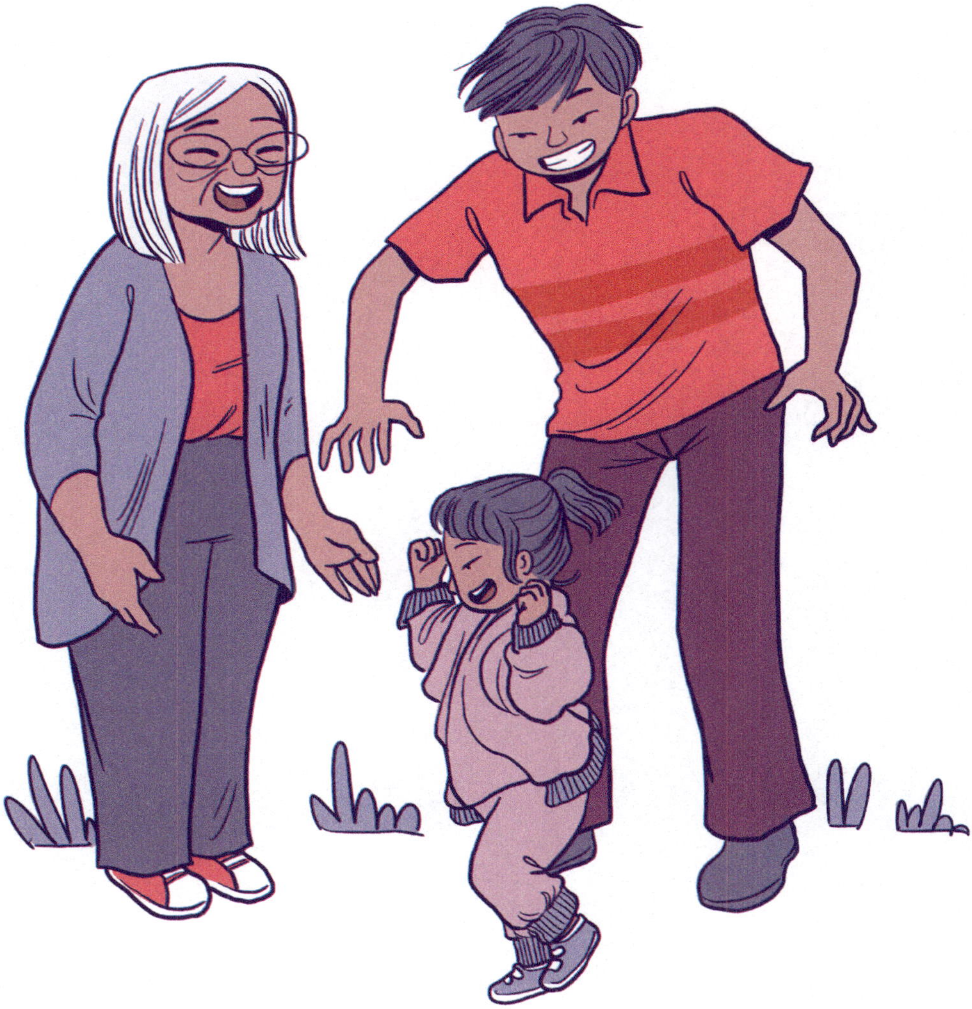

"Give us treats + sing songs" – GrandParents

This is a stage I have not yet reached but often ponder on how it will affect me. I don't want to wish my life away, or the kids', but seriously, I can't wait to be a nan, nanny, gran or grandma! I often wonder what kind of grandparents Steve and I will make – sounds very bizarre, I know!

I have been wondering for a while what angle I should go with for this chapter and have decided to go with my perspective, as I have done throughout the book. To get a grandparent's perspective, I have, like in all other chapters, got inspiration from fab grandparents. However, some of my 'spoonfuls of love' in this chapter are aimed at grandparents – as told by other grandparents. As they have been there they have 'walked the walk' and want to reach out to others.

Life with my own grandparents

I had six grandparents growing up, I had a great nan and grandad up until I was eight, then two sets of nanas and grandads for many years – my mum's parents and my dad's parents. It was only recently that my nan and grandad passed on my mother's side, with my nan and grandad playing a large part in my life, especially when growing up.

I am so grateful for having grandparents in my life and for my children having great grandparents for their early childhood. I have fond memories of sleepovers with my cousins at my nan and grandad's and often think of them now, remembering the great suppers we used to have and the card games we used to play.

My dad's dad was a baker so I always looked forward to a nice cake when we went to see them. Baking cakes is something that I always think about when I am a nan. I look forward to making special nan cakes for my grandchildren.

For some reason, my nanas and grandads were all named after their dogs! Nana and Grandad Candy and Nana and Grandad Meesa. I will have to get my mum and dad to explain that to me at some point! Not sure why I felt the need to mention this, but it still makes me chuckle.

Like me, my children still have two sets of grandparents and are extremely close to them all. Nanny Janice, Grandad George, Grandma and Grandad Ken. As I have mentioned earlier in this book, Steve and I are very grateful for the support that our parents have given us over the years. I have always wanted our parents to be included in our children's lives and we are lucky that we all live close together and all get on so well.

I do know that this is not always the case. I speak to many grandparents who find it a difficult relationship to maintain for many reasons: fractious relationship with daughter-in-law, not living close by, finding the children naughty, etc.

A special role

Being a grandparent can be a magical time. I read an article once saying being a grandparent has all the joys of being a parent without the responsibility – I think this sums it up well. I see this with our parents; the grandparents don't often get involved in the difficult conversations with grandchildren and are rarely the ones who give out discipline, leading to a nurturing and respectful relationship. I have seen over the years with friends that opinions given by grandparents have been the start of many arguments.

I am often shocked how often – particularly now my children are teens – that I go to my parents for parenting advice. I must admit I didn't think this was something that I would do but then I remember what I was like as a teen and that my parents got us all through this stage! It is always good advice and I am grateful for their listening ear. They are also good at staying quiet when not asked for advice.

"Don't offer parenting advice unless it's asked for. I hear from many mums who struggle with parenting comments made from mums/mums-in-law."

The gift of time

Time can be a difficult topic of conversation for many at this stage, with each generation viewing time in a different way. Depending on where we are in life, time can be seen very differently. In this chapter I explore what I mean by this. Obviously, everyone's circumstances are different but below is a trend that I see taking place for many families.

Time as viewed as a grandparent

For many grandparents at this stage in their life, there may be lots of other activities that they now do as a result of the benefits of the empty nest stage, but for many others these days can be long with few people to communicate with.

At times, grandparents may be torn as to how much they look after their grandchildren, sometimes feeling guilty if they are unable to or simply don't want to help. For many grandparents, this may be the opportunity to travel or see more friends. It can be a time that they want to make the most of their new-found freedom before they are unable.

Later in life, however, grandparents may stay longer and the days can be long with very little communication with others. Many older people that I know wait all day for a phone call from their children or wait all week for their family to visit them on the weekend, and can be disappointed when that visit or phone call doesn't take place.

Time as viewed as a parent

As mentioned throughout the book, we have been privileged to have family around who have helped a lot over the years with childcare, but this did come with us feeling indebted to them. Not that anything was ever said by our parents and I am sure they didn't feel this way, but it was certainly how I felt.

As our parents got older and illnesses started to arise, it was also important for us to realise when we needed to sort out our own child care to make sure we supported them more as well as give them a break from child care responsibilities. I must admit at times that checking in with grandparents has to be a conscious thought process because our weeks are so busy and one minute it's Monday the next it's Friday, with no communication with anyone in between.

One thing I have noticed from my own personal parenting journey compared to my parents' is the family working dynamic. For most families, it was the dads who had a job outside the home, and our mums were the ones who sorted out all the school activities, and kept the home running. For most nowadays there is far more of a joined-up approach with both parents working and the children doing far more activities, which can lead to parents not sitting down till late at night and only catching an hour a day to themselves. Leaving very little time for anything else in the week.

I know sometimes our parents need to be reminded what busy weeks we have. When their life has slowed down they may feel ignored, forgetting how busy life can be. However, it is equally important that we don't forget our parents are in need of communication and company.

A Sprinkle of Light to Lead the Way – Balancing the needs of everyone

- *If you have siblings, make sure you approach them to support you. For many it may be that your sibling is not local, but simply using them as a sounding board may help.*
- *Be realistic with what you can achieve, and also what you feel your parents can achieve as part of grandparent 'duties'.*
- *Close family time together can be precious. As I have mentioned throughout the book, time can go so fast and so it can be important to spend time together. You should not feel guilty about prioritising your time together. Explain to the older generations in your family why this time is so precious for you. I am sure they will understand as they have been there themselves.*

Time as viewed from a grandchild

Time for children, tweens and teens, as we know, is all about what they want to do when they want to do it. Teens especially spend a lot of time in their room and everything is an effort above and beyond leaving that room. So asking them to send a message to their grandparents or visiting them is like asking them to go to the moon and back! I will continue with the topic shortly.

The 'sharing of time'

More often than not, there seems to be one set of grandparents that are more involved with the children. This may be because of distance, but also can be because of overbearing grandparents or that one parent favours their own parents over their partners' parents.

From grandparents and parents that I have spoken with, this can be very distressing and causes lots of friction within the family. I have even known it to split couples up.

I have always tried to balance it out, especially as both our parents live locally and have a lot to do with each. It can be difficult at times to make sure you share your time and your children's time so that each set of grandparents gets an equal share of our time. It's like making sure you don't have a favourite child!

Relationship with grandchildren

This can be a tricky one! As well as spending time with grandparents, encouraging a nurturing and respectful relationship can be a tricky one! As children stop being looked after by their grandparents in the day, or don't see them when they are picked up from school, etc. – if they ever were – it can be difficult for them to see their grandparents, or should I say, want to see them!

Without the risk of making my children sound like spoiled little brats, in our household we have to remind them to come down and see their grandparents when they visit, and at times they do have to be forced to visit grandparents, asking every time, "Why do I have to go"?

Our children are at an age now that we can be quite blunt and tell them that their grandparents won't be here forever! Harsh, I know, but also the reality.

During Covid, however, there was a game changer. The children set up group chats on WhatsApp with their grandparents. Dylan was obviously too young but used ours. This has helped keep them in contact ever since and kept their grandparents involved in their daily lives, and also kept them up on technology! A total win, win situation.

A change in times

Over the years, undoubtedly the world has changed. A few sayings that I hear from one of our parents in particular are:

> *"back in the day"*
>
> *"the good old days"*
>
> *"happy days"*

Often referring to the way "the world has gone mad" (in their opinion).

The way that we talk and live our lives now is very different to when our parents were young. We live in a far more liberal world now and what is socially acceptable to say has changed. But this can be difficult for older generations when they have spent all their lives being able to say things that are no longer appropriate. I don't want to give an example in this book but I am sure you will all know what kind of sayings I mean.

My grandparents in particular would say inappropriate things about gender, sexuality and race. It used to upset me, but luckily my children were only young at the time and didn't understand the concept of the conversations.

At times now, some of our parents say comments that make my children look at Steve and I – but my children are now at an age where they understand that times have changed and what their grandparents say isn't always what they mean.

It's not for me to say how you should deal with situations like this. Your relationships with your parents/in-laws may be strong enough to challenge what they are saying, explaining that it is not appropriate anymore to say certain things. It may be easier to explain to your children that their grandparents use language that is no longer socially acceptable and they should not repeat what they hear! I tend to go with both scenarios, depending on what is being said and in what tone.

Keeping everyone involved happy

This can be very difficult and is one of the issues that has arisen many times over the years in my counselling room and groups that I have facilitated. From all that I have mentioned above, there is lots to consider and it is difficult to keep everyone happy.

So many individuals in the mix, spread over many generations, with individuals seeing situations quite differently. What I also find at this stage is that there is no changing anyone's opinions and the key to keeping everyone happy is compromise – that very difficult word, compromise! The problem lies when no one is willing to compromise – then arguments take place. I am afraid that I have no answers for this situation; I sure wish that I did.

Intergenerational relationships

I think that it is clear throughout this book that I have always been grateful to both sets of parents for their support throughout my own mothering journey. I know this is not the case for many and my heart always goes out to mums who have not got their own parents close by (this is starting to be more and more as families move away more now.) I also know many mums who have lost their parents and experience the huge loss that their passing creates. This takes me back to the start of my *Motherwell Cheshire* journey. The very reason I set up the charity was to create a community of women that support each other – much like the saying, 'It takes a village to raise a child.'

However, when it is possible to have access to the older generations in your family, or even with older people in your community, there are so many benefits for intergenerational support and I see this every day.

Grandparent relationships can be very special, and within the charity I see first-hand how intergenerational relationships can be precious. Different generations can learn from each other, the older generation offering wise words, the younger generation keeping the older young. Sharing stories and learning from each other brings value to both sides.

These intergenerational relationships don't mean that the people involved have to be related. In our groups, we see lots of strong relations form between women of all ages, with mutual respect for each other. All parties bring something special to the relationship.

Here, three grandparents share their special stories of being a grandmother, Gigi and Gran!

Life as Gigi – Ginette's Story

What is a Gran/Grandma/Nan/Nanny, or in my case, Gigi?

Growing up, my own gran, on my mum's side, had a huge presence in my life. I remember going to work with my mum on the bus and Gran meeting us to take me home with her while my mum worked. I also remember being at my Gran's a lot over the weekends along with my older brother and staying over often. I either went home or to my Gran's for lunch when I moved to high school; both meals which she would have made for me whether I was eating at home or at hers. When I was older, I would go back to her house between two and three in the morning when I had been out drinking. In short, her door was never closed, it was home from home. But in all those years she never seemed to change; she always lived in the same house, had the same routine and went to Bulgaria for two weeks once a year on a coach. She always seemed to be an old lady with a limp and grey hair in a beehive!

I am lucky enough to have a very close relationship with both of my daughters, so I have to admit that when my oldest daughter told me she was pregnant with my first grandchild, I had a lot of mixed emotions! I was too young, I was forty-six... just!!! My daughter was only twenty-two (I was only a year older when I had her), and since being nineteen, life had thrown her some fairly big curve balls. One of those curve balls was a health-related problem which had to be closely monitored throughout her pregnancy, resulting in her being hospitalised a couple of times. It was a big concern, both for my daughter and her unborn child.

My daughter asked me to be with her and her partner throughout the delivery of their daughter – one of the most amazing experiences I have ever witnessed.

However, again there were complications. My hours-old granddaughter was whisked off from her mum and dad to the Special Care Baby Unit (SCBU). In those first few days we didn't know what was wrong with her and she was tested for all sorts, including having to have a lumbar puncture. My daughter needed a blood transfusion, and I have to be honest, this tiny person rocked into our worlds and turned it upside down, leaving me feeling torn between the two of them – supporting my daughter and the worry and concern for my granddaughter. That worry for this little tornado who had arrived, I was trying not to show to my daughter. However, after a rollercoaster couple of days, my granddaughter was released from SCBU with a clean bill of health and came home.

I was always very protective of my daughters. I think it caught me a little off guard how this unconditional love and protectiveness automatically enveloped my granddaughter as well. It was a strange feeling in the early days to feel both concerned for my daughter and completely besotted with this little person, all at the same time trying to remember how I had managed to look after such a tiny thing myself as well as being mindful of giving mum and dad support and space. It felt like a real balancing act. She was their daughter, not mine. Where was my place? I hadn't figured that out yet, but at that time my place was wherever they needed me to be.

Two-and-a-half years later, granddaughter number two arrived into our world with no complications for her, but again resulted in emergency surgery and blood transfusions after the birth, for my daughter. This time I was at home looking after granddaughter number one, wondering if that unconditional love and protective bubble would stretch further again – it did!

My oldest granddaughter is five-and-a-half now, and her little sister is two-and-a-half. With the strong relationship I have with my daughters, I always expected to have a good relationship with my grandchildren. However, I don't think I expected to be quite so enmeshed in their everyday lives as I am.

I feel privileged every day that their parents trust me enough to drop off and pick them up from school and nursery, to take them off swimming or away for the weekend, to love them and chastise them when needed without question. I feel lucky to be able to see them most days without having to ask. It amazes me to watch these two completely different characters grow and learn, and watch their personalities develop. As Gigi, there is more time to take in everything they are saying and doing. They make me smile and laugh most days and sometimes they make me want to tear my hair out, but I would not change a second of it. And to top it all, the major bonus of being a Gigi is after a long day I also get to give them back! I suppose/hope being Gigi is very much like my own Gran was for me, a home from home, somewhere to be safe and know you are loved...but without the beehive!

Grandmothers – Joyce Williams' (aka Grandma Williams.com) story

Yes, I am a grandmother with two grandsons, though both now over thirty. That sweet cuddly, charming, tiring stage is long over. We have gone past adventurous exploring, fun holidays and teenage agonies. They have become my friends and advisors and I hope I theirs. We share life's understandings and concerns as adults and I learn technology from them.

Looking back, as one does with interest at eighty-eight, I have decided to talk about the bigger role of grandmothers. That of us being 'living history'.

My own grandmother was born in 1870 – that makes me the holder of 150 years of life memories, from Victorian to new Carolinian. It struck me forcibly on bonfire night that we were sitting listening to explosions with pleasure and prosecco whilst in Gaza children were hearing similar noises with terror. And I was the only one amongst us who knew what that experience was actually like. I too had cowered in a shelter with sirens and bombs overhead, Mother cradling us and Dad out in it all, firefighting. We heard the planes coming over and the whoosh before the bang and knew the relief that it wasn't us this time. Seeing familiar streets and buildings in ruins and playing on bomb sites were normal. As was rationing. Clothes rationing was the worst. We grew our own veg, so we always had food. And afterwards, the hopeless lack of housing.

It was looking back on the scale of change in my own life and that of my grandmothers that made me realise how different our perspective is from that of our grandchildren. And perhaps how valuable it is to be able to see that longer view.

For example, both my grandmothers had illegitimate babies in their lives. Note that word! Not really in use today is it? Illegitimacy was a disgrace. One grandmother 'took in' my mother, who was her friend's illegitimate baby – being a single mother then was not an option. My grandmother had recently lost a premature baby, so all this was done quite informally.

My mother was not told until she was about to get married herself and had to know her real name. At which point she told my father she couldn't let him have the disgrace of marrying a bastard. Luckily, he said "Rubbish!" But it wasn't society's opinion. They had to move and marry in a Registry office so the banns wouldn't be read in their town. My mother had to tell me when I needed my birth certificate for my 11+ exam, totally distressed to admit that she was a bastard even in 1945. I was sworn not to tell.

It is hard to understand that society. My other grandmother almost certainly 'had to get married' (and we think not to the father of her child) to save her name. I have her wedding nightdress. White linen, high frilled neck, buttoned up and long sleeves, which says much about sexual attitudes then.

What moral view that we hold today will be completely changed in our grandchildren's lives? I suspect that, like back then, they can't imagine anything different. But then in my grandmother's time, homophobia was rife. And the death sentence was normal as was the workhouse.

When you are living in a specific period you can't imagine that your beliefs and understandings will be judged very differently by later generations.

Millions of homes missing after the war, living with in-laws the norm. We did recognise the need for social housing and got on with it. Expect we shall again.

Living through the polio epidemic taught us the importance of vaccines. Maybe it is up to grandmothers to remind this generation of the awful consequences diphtheria, measles, etc. brought in our pre-vaccine childhoods. My grandmother had a severe prolapse. No treatment, was told "no more children", but no easy contraception. As she told my mother: "I was lucky I had a considerate husband."

Health changes have been truly amazing and will continue. If I were eighty-eight in my grandmothers' time, I would now be blind with cataracts, deaf, no teeth and definitely an arthritic cripple. Our NHS and joint replacements have transformed old age.

Women must have been so tough in my grandmothers' time. My grandmother had a working husband – a travelling blacksmith – but she had to take in laundry to make ends meet. Up early to carry the coal and light the fire to heat the copper. Fill it with buckets of water. Boil, soak and pound the white washing, pull out, wring and rinse in a washtub. Dirty stuff in next, plus significant scrubbing on a washboard. Make starch, boil more water for starching shirts, collars and linens. Haul out and put through a heavy manual wringer. My grandmothers had wooden rollers which broke the pearl shirt buttons, so another job was to replace those later. Hang out to dry if not wet, or around a fire if it rains. Hoping soot wouldn't drop on whites. Next day, iron with coal heated iron, and mend, then lump clean laundry baskets back to owners.

Always kneading bread and carrying shopping daily, plus full chamber pots taken carefully down to outdoor loo. Never needed to go to a gym to get fit!

We tend to look back at Victorians and think how could they have allowed poverty like that? Why did they pollute the air and rivers? And have such unforgiving moral values?

My challenge to you for our grandchildren is to allow them to see this long perspective. And ask themselves what their great grandchildren will think of their values and actions.

How will they excuse using plastics and ultra-processed foods, for example? And will their moral values stand up to 150 years of scrutiny?

Being a nana – Debbie's story

Where do I start...? I had two wonderful nanas in my life, Big Nana and Little Nana. So called because one was a big lady and the other very slight and frail. Big Nana was my mum's mum and we saw more of her, staying with her during the holidays in Salford. I probably felt closer to her and have lots of fond memories. The food she prepared: pea and ham soup, cold fresh orange juice off the milkman, Rice Krispies and tiny Hovis loaves of bread. Fond memories of waking up on Christmas morning in her house and being allowed to go to the paper shop on my own to fetch the Manchester Evening News and my tiny Hovis loaf. She spoilt me rotten and I loved it! It's what nanas do! Little Nana we saw less often. She lived in Manchester and my memory was of a house less homely. Both nanas died when I was about ten years old. They were around seventy-five but I remember they always seemed old. I watched my Big Nana die slowly from cancer as she came to live with us. We were all devastated. Not only did I lose my nanas but I lost my connections to Manchester, where I was born. We seldom returned.

When I was twenty-eight and then again at thirty I had my girls and my mum stepped into the nana shoes. She was fifty-eight and adored them, making sure she saw them as often as she could, probably every two weeks as we lived a good hour's drive away and she was still working. We often stayed there and my girls still remember her house, and in particular the smells. Sadly, she died when I was thirty-five and she was sixty-five, so my girls lost their nana very early on and Jonny never got to meet her. Despite only being a nana for seven years, she left a massive void in our lives and, for me, a huge expectation to fill. How could I ever be a s good as her as a nana?

In April 2019, my daughter Hannah, announced that she was pregnant, due in December, really close to my other daughter's birthday. I lived every second with her, enjoying the photos of her tummy growing, news of scans, the sex of the baby – a boy!!

George Rodney arrived early on 5th December and I had to wait a whole day before I could see them. I was fifty-eight and ready to take on the challenge! Poor Hannah had a rough time. I was worried sick about her as news was slow coming through. I wasn't at George's birth, which I'm probably glad about as I don't think I could've stood watching Hannah go through the pain – he was ten pounds!

Hannah really struggled for the first few months and I was sad when she asked her in-laws to support them in the first few weeks. We've talked about it since and I understand her rationale. This took us into the pandemic with Covid-19. However, I came into my own when six months later, just as we were coming out of lockdown, Hannah really started to struggle with her mental health. She hadn't dealt with a traumatic birth and we believe she was probably suffering from post-traumatic stress disorder. Luckily, I was able to stay with her and support her as she really didn't believe she was able to look after George. She got through it and is now a far better mum than I ever was. I'm so proud of her!

Compared to many of my friends, I was quite late becoming a nana and they all said, "Oh, you wait! There's nothing like the feeling you have for your grandchildren!" I could never imagine loving another child as much as I do my own three children, but this love is all encompassing; it took me by surprise!

It is a very different relationship to being a mum. I can spoil him, and overindulge him because I'm very aware that our time is precious. I want him to remember me with fondness, as being that crazy nana who'd do daft things with him. But the biggest drawback is not having the stamina to keep up with him – up at 5am Christmas morning AND Boxing Day saw me having a 'nana nap' to survive! I'd never have got up and stayed up that early normally, but that little voice breaking through my sleep, "Nana!" is irresistible! How can I say no as he dives into bed with me with his bunny, monster trucks and Spidermen? Only to be followed by book after book to read. . . .

George is now four, and very much like his mummy! Same beautiful big brown eyes, curly brown hair and initially shy and recent nature. But boy, when he warms to you, the trust you feel is so privileged as you know you've earned it! He trusts me to pick him up from nursery, he loves going in nana's car, going to the cafe to get treats for us and mummy and daddy, putting him to bed and reading his favourite bedtime book AND taking him to the toilet, joy of joys!

School is next. Time is going so quickly, but I'm looking forward to the next chapter of being George's Nana.

Reflections

There is the potential to be so many special moments being a grandparent, but this can come with many complications when family dynamics come into play. Prioritising the needs of everyone involved – your own children, your grandchildren and yourself – can become a struggle. Good, honest communication is key.

If you're reading this book and you're a parent with teens, like me, and balancing time between spending time with your children, time with your partner and time with your own parents, it can be a struggle and there is no right answer to balancing it all. Again, good communication between everyone makes it all go much more smoothly.

This stage is a stage that reminds me of memories, family memories that can be cherished by everyone.

"Make time to make memories."

Websites and helpful phone numbers:

Age UK: https://www.ageuk.org.uk

Gransnet: A website for grans! – https://www.gransnet.com

CBBC: For play inspiration – https://www.bbc.co.uk/tiny-happy-people/grandparents

Family lives: For advice and guidance – https://www.familylives.org.uk/advice/your-family/grandparents

Kinship Support: A charity that supports Kinship parents – https://kinship.org.uk

Final reflections

It has taken me years to write this book and I am so glad that it did in the end as it gave me an opportunity to experience another 'two stages' of the mothering journey.

My final reflections for this book is that for the majority of the stages, the practical and the emotional struggles mums may experience are the same but for different reasons.

We can be short of time with a newborn due to feeding and nappy changes, the same as being short of time with a teenager who needs lifts and support with after-school activities.

Women can lack libido when they have just given birth, the same as when they are going through the menopause.

Mum guilt follows us FOREVER at every stage of motherhood. I have experienced mum guilt and this is a theme in every chapter of my book.

In most cases in the book the 'A Spoonful of Love' and 'A Sprinkle of Light to Lead the Way' contributions could be attributed to any stage of the mothering journey. I do hope this book is a book that you pick up time and time again to help you on your mothering journey – it's what I envision the book is all about.

Thank you so much for taking the time to read my book. I hope that you have found the book honest and supportive.

I would love to connect with you and to hear your own stories and tips on this mad, crazy yet so fulfilling journey that is motherhood. Please feel free to get in touch with me:

Instagram: @mumstheword

Facebook: @Kate Blakemore Women and Girls Champion

Website: www.kateblakemore.co.uk

Twitter: @motherwellCEO

YouTube: Kate Blakemore

LinkedIn: Kay Blakemore

About the Author - Kate Blakemore

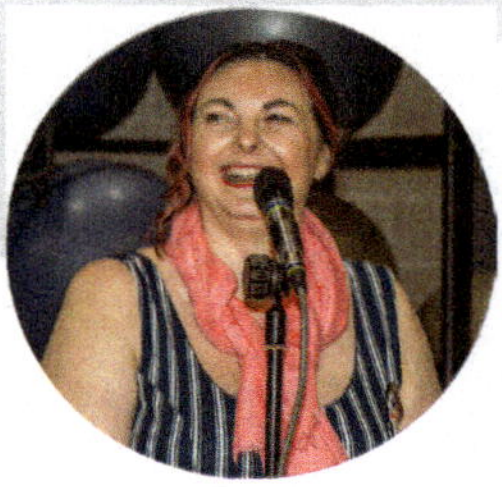

Kate Blakemore is a mum of three, who is a counsellor with specialism in infant loss and birth trauma. Kate has had her private counselling practice since 2012 and has a diploma in Specialist Fertility Counselling.

Kate is also the founder and Chief Executive of the charity *Motherwell Cheshire*, a Women and Girls charity which was founded in 2015.

Kate is passionate about supporting women and girls, and in particular mums' mental health. Kate felt there were many books out there for new mums but nothing really available for the mothering journey, and so the start of the book *Mum's the word – The Mothering Journey* began.

Thank you's

There are so many people that I need to thank for making this book possible so here goes…

Firstly, I would like to thank my fab editor and book mentor, Siân-Elin Flint-Freel, who has supported me so much on this journey, and kept me motivated every step of the way, as well as keeping me focused. I especially love that Siân-Elin was as excited as I was about my Mary Poppins quotes.

A big thank you to illustrator Carol Rossini for her artwork throughout this book. I am sure you will agree it is just amazing.

Thank you, Michelle Catanach, who designed my front cover and layout of the book. Thank you for your patience. I love each and every page.

I also cannot thank you enough, Nicola, Emma, Natalie, Emma, Lisa, Kate, Debb, Ginette, Melanie, Shelia, Leeanne, Cheryl, Caroline, Kirsten, Lorna, Danielle, Kirsty, Nic, and those who remain anonymous, for your contributions to this book.

I would also like to say a big heartfelt thank you to all the mums, the women who have formed part of my community over the years. These communities being our Motherwell Community and also my counselling community – your strength and resilience amazes me every day.

To the passionate, hardworking and inspiring *Motherwell Cheshire* team, our charity simply wouldn't be the same without each and every one of you.

Finally, thank you to my loyal friends and family who have supported me every step of the way.

Printed in Great Britain
by Amazon

48621596R00126